Running with the Girls

Lacie Whyte
and
Dane Rauschenberg

Contents

FOREWORD IX

INTRODUCTION 1

1 - HISTORY OF WOMEN'S RUNNING 3

2 - PAM RICKARD 11

3 - MEAGAN NEDLO 19

4 - KRIS GRACI 29

5 - HEATHER ALVARADO 37

6 - MICHELLE WALKER 45

7 - MYLA JOHNSON 55

8 - ANNIE BURKE 65

9 - WOMEN'S RUNNING TODAY 73

10 - HOLLY KOESTER 79

11 - LAURA FREY 87

12 - MICHELLE NIEMEYER, LAURA HILEMAN AND SHANNON
MITCHEL 95

13 - LUISA MILLER 105

14 - BREEZY BOCHENEK 113

15 - CAMILLE HERRON 121

16 - SOPHIA SHI 129

17 - MONIKA ALLEN 137

18 - WHERE CAN WE GO FROM HERE? 147

To Hailey,

My biggest inspiration of all.

"Once I passed through that tunnel,
I knew things would never be the same."
— Joan Benoit

Foreword

The glossy covers of my favorite running magazines feature running heroes: Olympians, Boston Marathon winners, and professional athletes. Sometimes the magazines look back at the pioneers of our sport who blazed the trail and opened doors for us all. Often they are today's elite runners. Without a doubt, these women should be celebrated and highlighted. At the same time, I find myself wondering why we don't see more women featured or honored who lack sponsorship dollars, lucrative shoe contracts or the DNA that allows either of those to happen. Those women who have a deep love of running, and are getting it done solely for their own reasons and drive rarely get the same press. I'm talking about the runner next door or the one you see on your favorite trail each morning. You don't know her name or where she works but you understand her implicitly. You have a connection and kinship.

Realizing this bond exists and not seeing what I felt was what women truly hoped to see in their running publications, it became a dream of mine to write a book dedicated to them. Dedicated to you. After participating in variety of races across the country and meeting countless dynamic women along the way, I knew I had to grab the horse by the reins and make that book happen.

When I first set out on this adventure to write a book, it never occurred to me how engulfed I would become in the extraordinary lives of these women runners. I have had the distinct pleasure of interacting with them over multiple interviews and meetings. I became very connected to their stories and lives; remaining that way months after our interviews have wrapped. I could not help but be incredibly moved by learning what running means to these women. Their tales include their own special journeys involving children, careers, marriages, divorces, weight loss, illness and how they coped with the many curveballs thrown at them. Which can be relentless at times. When I could put myself into their shoes and realized all of these struggles could happen to me and many other women, I became even more resolved to share each and every one of them.

The vulnerability the women featured in this book showed, and the strength they have in allowing us to interview them, has made me strive to be a better person and friend. They continue to inspire me each time I re-read their chapters. Long after the conversations were over I kept thinking of one word to describe how these women were: brave. Brave to share, brave to put themselves out there, brave to be so authentic, so open.

Most of the women come from completely different backgrounds, thousands of miles apart, but the common factor that intertwined them all was running. For some it was how the sport helped them through a particularly difficult time. For others running made them feel more confident about themselves. Finally, and this resonated with me the most, running showed these women they could achieve something they never thought possible. Whether that achievement was a 5k or their first ultra or nothing to do with running at all, they pushed passed previous set limitations. They did so, almost always, by nothing more than sheer will.

Sheer will I understand. Running, however is something that came later to me in life. While I was consistently involved in athletics throughout high school, most involved team sports. I never really 'got' running. I heard of people speaking about the runners' high or really hitting their stride after getting six miles under their belt and I thought they were, well, crazy.

An injury, which sidelined a collegiate athletic career, led me to running in the first place. However, it was hardly love at first fartlek. I didn't really fall in love with the sport, however, until I went through my divorce in 2008. Emotionally I was at my lowest point. I simply felt like a failure. I needed to find a way out of this darkness, but battled the deep-rooted fear of not knowing how to get myself out.

My daughter was only three at the time and I realized that I had to somehow pull myself out of the despair I was experiencing. I had to be a strong example for her and desperately needing a way out of my sadness. I didn't know it then, but signing up for a half marathon was the best thing I could have done for myself. There was something therapeutic about writing my training schedule down in my moleskin calendar. Spreadsheets and the internet are nice but I still love the act of writing and having a physical paper calendar to refer to. Having my training schedule in black and white, crossing off workouts as I completed them, gave me the feeling of accomplishment. Little by little, I found myself again. I finally understood what those idiotic runners were talking about. To this day, no matter what life throws at me, a nice long run makes everything more tolerable.

That is why I hope you enjoy these remarkable life stories as much as I do. I have no doubt you will draw your own inspiration from them. We each have our own unique experience and everyone has his or her own journey to share. Within every one of us lies a passion for something and I love the fact that this book connects us to each other, because of our shared love of running.

So, celebrate and relish the lives of everyday women runners you know who somehow balance their chaotic schedules and running. Celebrate how fabulous they are. Then in turn, and, most importantly, celebrate yourselves.

Introduction

When Lacie approached me with the idea of collaborating on a book which chronicled the stories of inspirational women, I loved the idea. My one caveat was that the women we profiled had to cut a swath through a larger portion of the general female experience. While the stories which headline magazines or are fodder for the big screen are wonderful, they are a tad unrelatable. In addition, including only the extreme ends of inspiration turned a blind eye to what other women who, on a daily basis, do. These tales might be a little less incredible but are still extremely moving. Fortunately, Lacie was on the exact same page.

Without a doubt this book will feature women who have overcome both trauma and strife. In addition, it will make sure to highlight women who have succeeded in a variety of different ways, which often fly under the radar. We want to show how the small battles won each day add to the major wars being won down the road. Furthermore, even if setbacks occur in your life, and they will, they tend not to be the end of the line for you. Overcoming trouble is something we can all do even if we fall behind here and there.

The greatest and worst thing about running is that it is participatory. This means more people take part in running and racing than any other activity in America. The bad part of that is because so many are participating they often do not look at the history of the sport and how we got to where we are. We have remedied just a sliver of that problem by shining a light on where women have come from in running, where they are today, and where we expect them to be in the future.

This book will also address a problem we feel is rather rampant in the coverage of the sport of running. The women profiled in this book cover all ages, races, religions, abilities and levels of hardship. However, if you look at the cover of prominent running publications, you would think that there are only a small handful of women in which you can either learn from or pay attention to. While we love reading the stories of the women at the top of this sport, knowing more about those at all levels, in all disciplines, in all distances makes us not only more well-rounded in our knowledge of women runners but as historians of where we have come. We need to realize how lucky we are to be in this sport where we are.

I say "we" because men too are extremely lucky women have been part of the history of running, most prominently in the last thirty years or so. The changes and innovations, not to count the sheer number of bodies taking on racing, have moved us all forward in leaps and bounds.

If you are hoping to be moved by multiple tales of women who are some of the most relatable you have ever read about, then be glad this book is in your hands. And if you can keep yourself from lacing up your shoes and going for a run after reading it, then there might not be a cure for your non-running-itis.

1

History of Women's Running

If you are a woman under thirty years of age, the chances are high you are not aware of how just a few short decades ago, the opportunities to participate in many sports simply did not exist for you. This lack of knowing is a good thing. It means the work of the people who came before you was done thoroughly. If you cannot fathom not being able to play a sport simply because you had breasts, then those pioneers did not toil in vain. However, we cannot forget to remember that so much which we have today, especially in the sport of running, comes from women pioneers of this sport. Not knowing where we have come from is a not only a great disservice to ourselves but a slap in the face to those women who did what they did so we can do what we do.

As such, while this book will be sharing many wonderful stories of the women who are showing us what they can do today, it is best to start with just a skimming of the background of women's running so we know what was done to get us here.

The 1960 Summer Olympics in Rome are remembered for many things in the world of running. Most famously,

Abebe Bikila of Ethiopia won the marathon running barefoot. You can see why it took some visionaries just forty odd years to kick-start a barefoot running craze. (Intense sarcasm intended.) However, Bikila's victory there and again four years later in Mexico City (wearing shoes) helped launched what decades later would be an African dominance in the marathon. Yet, it is a lesser-known turn of event that really changed the culture of running worldwide. Women athletes, for the first time, were allowed to participate in five separate running events in the Summer Olympics. While this total was still less than the sixteen races open to men in those same Olympics, it heralded a change for women athletics of every kind.

Women have historically been seen as the more frail gender. While there are obviously differences between the two sexes, virtually all of the reasoning behind thinking women need to be coddled is either based on conjecture, falsehood or just outright sexism. However, in the world of running, it did not necessarily start out this bad.

In the 1928 Summer Olympics in Amsterdam, women raced very hard in, amongst other things, the 800-meter run, for the first time in Olympic history. One would think that the fact that this happened over 80 years ago would signify people of the time were more progressive than the next several decades with regards to women's liberation. However, these efforts were not without protest by many. Also, it would be the last time for years women were allowed to do so.

Press reports of the 800-meter run claimed that many of the competitors were exhausted or failed to finish the race.

Stories were told of women collapsing at the finish line, bereft of oxygen and energy. Lolling around on the ground, some reportedly were close to death. At best having women compete in such a way was unladylike; at worst, it was horrific display of an inferior gender. It's also too bad that such a thing never actually happened.

A thorough examination of the evidence from the day, including eyewitness accounts and newspaper reports, tell quite a different story. Nine women entered the 800-meter finals on race day. All nine not only completed the race standing up but several bettered the existing world's record. In fact, when all was said and done, none of the women were even unnaturally winded. Without a doubt there was no exhaustion or near-death displays. Any report of the frailty of female competitors was absolute malarkey. Unfortunately, there were no cell phone cameras or twitter to stem the tide of false information. The damage was done. Almost immediately women's running events of any length longer than 200 meters were removed from international competition.

It wasn't until these historic 1960 Olympics that women were once allowed to run half of a mile in competition. This ignored the fact that women had been running many miles longer on their own in training and had actually completed marathon distances themselves. Yet, this small step was at least a step forward. It laid the groundwork for where women's running would go in the near future. Well, not the near near future. But not 2037 either, thankfully.

You see in 1961, the Amateur Athletic Union (AAU) banned women from competing officially in all U.S. road races. If you don't know your history, trust us in saying that the AAU was simply one of the worst things ever created (worse than Crystal Pepsi. Wait. You don't know what that is either? You kids with your Angry Birds and your Justin Bieber, I tell ya.) To put it simply, the AAU banned women from competing in any capacity, kept all male runners from making any semblance of living under the guise of "amateurism" and basically allowed stodgy old men to make backroom deals to better themselves and themselves alone. This was presumably done covered in cigar smoke, with lots of backslapping and deep-resonating evil laughter while they lit $100 bills and threw them at puppies. There is no proof of this happening but there is no proof they didn't either.

Cartoonish attempts to paint the picture of the AAU aside, it was a horrible organization. Even when statements were attempted to be made by women to show what they could do, the press would still find a way to marginalize them and sexualize them. A nineteen-year-old runner named Julia Chase entered a 6.5-mile road race in Chicopee, Massachusetts in 1961, attempting to challenge the ban. She garnered some attention for taking part in the race but was largely treated as a spectacle. One report stated: "Miss Chase said she is 5'4", weighs 118 pounds and does not know her other dimensions. (Eyewitnesses report her other dimensions are very good.)" We are not making this up. Chase ended up beating right of the men running that day. There are no confirmed reports of any of the men having their uterus fall out.

Now, any runner worth their salt, especially women runners who now get to run unfettered by any gender bias, should know who Kathrine Switzer is and her contributions to the sport. We will get to her groundbreaking achievements soon. But this book wants to give you even more knowledge of the trailblazers out there. One in particular is Bobbi Gibb.

Bobbi simply wanted to run the Boston Marathon. She had put in the miles and the sweat for two years in order to be able to do so. In February 1966, upon sending in a letter asking for an application to the race (there were not qualifying times yet) she received a letter from the race director, Will Cloney, informing her that women were not physiologically capable of running marathon distances. Undeterred, after hiding in the bushes and jumping into the race at the start, Bobbi went on to show the ludicrous nature of that notion. Her efforts did not go unnoticed. It didn't take long for the press to pick up news of a female running in the race. With just a few hundred participants running it wasn't hard to see her. By the time Gibb reached the finish line in Boston, the Governor of Massachusetts, John Volpe, was there to shake her hand. Given she finished in 3:21:42 and ahead of two-thirds of the pack, it is a wonder the Governor even had time to make it there. Yet even this effort was considered quaint at best.

Gibb had made a statement but it was a quiet one. It was one that allowed her to get a handshake and be pleasantly ignored afterward. Her competitors on the course were almost, to the person, supportive of her efforts. The crowds went wild when she ran by. Yet, nothing of note changed for the rest of female running population. They were still ignored and marginalized. So Gibb decided to return the next year and ran again. She finished nearly an hour ahead of

Kathrine Switzer. But fortunately, for all of us, Kathrine had raised the ire of Jock Semple.

Switzer ran the 1967 Boston Marathon with an official bib by registering under the name K.V. Switzer. This, according to Switzer was not a ruse to get pass the AAU ban but rather something she commonly used to sign papers. She, like Gibb, simply wanted to run the race she had trained so hard for. She had already run longer than 26.2 miles in one training session and knew it was possible. She just had to do it.

Having women showboating in the race and getting attention from the mayor like Gibb did was one thing. But a female having an official bib was far too much for Jock Semple, the curmudgeonly overseer of all things Boston Marathon. When he jumped off the press truck and tried to remove Switzer's number, he was body-blocked by Switzer's hammer-throwing college athlete boyfriend. Unlike fluff pieces told third-handedly, this entire spectacle happened right in front of the entire media. Pictures were taken and quickly made the rounds to the papers. Women's running, through the tireless efforts of so many pioneers, was finally beginning to get the attention it deserved. Well, again, "beginning" is a relative word. Switzer was banned from by the AAU. Yet given the AAU had already banned her, we are guessing this had little effect on her decision to run.

When the AAU finally progressed pass Cro-Magnon thinking and allowed women to register for marathons, they still did so in underhanded, conniving, backhanded ways (Seriously – you should hate the AAU even though it doesn't exist anymore.) Stating that women had to start at a separate time or starting line than men, the AAU prompted the women of the 1972 New York City Marathon to protest. Sitting down at the starting line, legs crossed in defiance, they simply waited for 10 minutes until the men's gun went off. Then away they went.

As the 1970s moved on, women were not just running races, being defiant and posting "nice" times. They were running fast and hard. In 1979, Grete Waitz became the first woman in history to finish 26.22 miles in less than two and a half hours by shattering her own world record in a time of 2:27:33. Fortunately, a year later, the American College of Sports Medicine released a statement in support of the creation of the women's Olympic Marathon. It stated:

"There exists no conclusive scientific or medical evidence that long-distance running is contraindicated for the healthy, trained female athlete."

I bet Grete and the thousands of women who had been running long-distance for years were relieved to know they were not competing in some Matrix-esque world. Way to be on top of things, ACSM.

In 1984, all those women pioneers we mentioned and so many more finally broke down the Olympic walls. The Women's Marathon makes its debut in the Los Angeles Summer Olympics that year. In the midst of the Cold War, with Russia boycotting the games, it definitely did not hurt the narrative that American runner Joan Benoit took home the gold. There is no better encapsulation of what this victory would mean to the future of women's running that what Joan said herself:

"Once I passed through that tunnel, I knew things would never be the same."

But it was not just women long-distance runners, or even professionals, who were vanguards of this change. In 1987, Jackie Joyner-Kersee appeared on the cover of Sports Illustrated, not in some frilly or posed way, but rather while chucking a javelin with all her muscular glory. Five years later, Gail Devers helps take down the idea that women can't be athletic and feminine at the same time when she wins the 100-meter dash with a fabulously flashy manicure. Two years after that, at the age of 40, Oprah Winfrey crosses the finish line at the Marine Corps Marathon after dropping more than 80 pounds. "Running is the greatest metaphor for life," the now littler O said, "Because you get out of it what you put into it."

Now, finally, without a doubt, the tide of women runners, wearing tutus and skirts, or bun huggers and sports bras, sweating and spitting and challenging themselves, was crashing down upon the world.

No, seriously, you should still be angry with the AAU.

2

Pam Rickard

We have all had bad days. Many of us are aware of how hard life can kick us when we are down. A few of us are unlucky enough (or is it lucky?) to know when we have hit bottom.

Pam Rickard knows where her rock bottom was.

Surprisingly, rock bottom was not the time she was walking from a liquor store with wine in a bag when she was supposed to be exercising at the YMCA. It didn't occur when her daughter drove up next to her begging her to get in the car and she kept on walking. After she had her third DUI arrest in an 18-month period when she knows she could have had thirty others she still had further to go. Even when that final DUI led to a three-month prison sentence, she was still not at rock bottom. No, it was when she could no longer literally look at herself in the mirror that she finally hitting bedrock. She had reached the point where she averted her gaze from her own reflection, as the lies were evident in her eyes. Unable to look into her own face, Pam Rickard found herself and knew change was needed.

Pam is, according to herself, a born alcoholic. She had her first drink when she was barely a teenager at tender age of fourteen. In high school, she was a social butterfly using alcohol to lubricate the wheels of popularity. She enjoying smoking and virtually all the things one can pictures happening in a 1970s high school. She most assuredly was not a runner. No, running would mean she would have to reapply her make-up or sweat a little bit. For Pam, life was about enjoying the here and now and enjoying it with as much alcohol as possible.

The biggest problem with Pam's drinking and obviously alcoholism was not that she was weak or a victim. In fact it was the opposite. Pam was then and is now made of tough material. She is, as they call it, a "highly-functioning" alcoholic. Unlike the fall-down drunks and slurring buffoons like Barney in the Simpsons, Pam put back the drinks and made it through life. She could do it clandestinely without many really knowing how much alcohol was in her system. She made it through high school that was quite easily. Then she moved onto college.

Pam decided to start studying journalism at Ohio University, a school tucked away in the hills of Athens, Ohio. The fact that OU is also known to be one of the biggest party schools in the nation didn't help Pam situation very much. Granted, Pam didn't need much encouragement to drink. In fact, the first race that Pam ran was a Homecoming 5k race in college, which she ran still drunk from a party that ended barely a few hours previously. She found the race tolerable and perhaps she might like this running thing. Well, as long as it didn't get in the way of drinking, though. Training would never take precedence over alcohol. The two might coincide but the former would never be more important than the latter.

So she would run here and there, taking part in some races locally. However it wasn't until graduation and accepting a job at the Pittsburgh Press did Pam begin to find the runner within her.

Routes around her home and work became treasured paths. After years of being one of the crowd she was now "Pam, the runner." She now had a separate personality and an identity all her own. Her running distances increased and she became a marathoner. Unfortunately, running also became an enabler for her drinking addiction. It would be impossible to be both an alcoholic and a person who runs 26.2 miles for fun, she thought. The marathon is far too grueling and difficult of an event to bring anything less than the best version of yourself to the line. One can't have a disease and conquer it. Obviously, she was just a social drinker. But man could she socially drink.

After dinner when everyone else was drinking is where Pam would throw down the chardonnay. As with many other women with drinking problems, Pam realizes she romanticized the nature of her alcoholism with wine. Men often take to beer or hard liquor that leaves clinking bottles rolling around on the floor as evidence. Wine, on the other hand, is classy and sophisticated. Plus, as an added bonus, with its higher value, wine allows more alcohol to be consumed with less empties lying around as proof of the problem. Win-win!

Pam married her college sweetheart and found her way to Roanoke Virginia, with a stable life and a few children. There were no outward signs of the problems that raged beneath. She exceeded at every job she had. Her drinking blackouts were just side effects of life. They were merely another thing she could handle, like shin splints or exhaustion at mile 45 of an ultramarathon. She didn't necessary wear her drinking as badges of honor but it wasn't a problem she needed with which she needed to bother herself or anyone else.

The one important time Pam did not drink was when she was pregnant with her children. She knew alcohol wasn't good for a baby even if she had a problem realizing how bad it was for her in the quantities she consumed. She also did not imbibe when she was breastfeeding. When she was in the nitty gritty of marathon training, she also was a teetotaler. Seven marathons were completed and three children born where alcohol took a backseat nursing or fartlek's. If only she ran more marathons or had more children, maybe she would have stopped drinking all together.

Instead, she was swirling in a perfect storm of arrogance and fear. There was an intense hopelessness to her life. While sometimes she rationalized her drinking, other times she clearly saw what a horrible problem she had. She was exhausted from putting on a façade of health when she was really killing herself. As the toll became greater she saw only two choices: taking her own life or surrendering to help. Fortunately, the first never happen. Unfortunately, for the longest time she never tried the latter either. Pam figured she was unfixable. She had drunk too hard, for too long to stop now. But when that third DUI finally put her into jail, she saw she no longer had a choice. She surrendered.

It was a normal Monday morning when Pam found herself driving to the Farley Center, the place she would seek help for her addiction. Well, it was normal if you aren't a runner. You see, Monday April 17th, 2006 was also the day of the Boston Marathon. Listening on the radio in silence with her husband as they drove to her saviors, Pam heard the radio talking about the Boston Marathon. She had actually qualified for the race numerous times but had never actually run it. Now instead of toeing the line at Hopkinton, she was going to alcohol rehab treatment center. She was no longer Pam the runner. She was Pam the alcoholic.

Her time at the center went by without much incident. For almost the entirety of her stay, Pam kept thinking back to that radio broadcast she heard about the Boston Marathon. She realized her running had not been about anything more than starting and finishing as fast as she could. She took for granted how lucky she was and had abused her body with alcohol through virtually all of her training save a few weeks here and there. When she checked out of the Farley Center she knew she wanted to run one more marathon. She had never run a marathon with "an integrity or authenticity". So she entered the 2007 NYC Marathon envisioning what running a big race would feel like without the effects of alcohol ravaging her body.

In the entry form for the NYC Marathon there is a spot where they ask you to share your story. Pam decided to tell a little bit about herself hoping maybe she could make a difference. Little did she know her story would become part of the book on the Marathon called 'A Race like No Other.' In fact, when she got the call to talk about her experiences, it was the first time anyone outside of her immediate family or her counselors got to hear the torment and self-inflicted pain she had gone through.

Pam never expected that little comment box to blossom into the next phase of her life. The book was a great success and Pam's part in it saw her soon back in rehab. This time, however, in a much different capacity. She would now be doing what she could to help those who traveled down the same path that she had and hopefully helping many others before they got that far.

She ended up with a brand new career when she was hired by the treatment center where she found her foundation for recovery. Or in her own words: "When I checked into the Farley Center, they took my cell phone. Now they pay for it." Working at what she describes as her dream job she serves as the VP Marketing for Runwell, The Linda Quirk Foundation. Yet even with this position, Pam knew she was not out of the woods. Every day she fights her addiction and knows she is just one bottle away from returning to that rock bottom once again. Pam is just a few sips away from where even the sight of her own face was unbearable. This knowledge that she is just as susceptible to the horrors of alcoholism drives her every day to help others.

Eight years have passed since that day she spent listening to the Boston Marathon and embarking on what would be the biggest change of her life. The challenges remain but Pam has taken the tenacity with which she used to hide her problems for so long and channeled it elsewhere.

Her dream job led to her running a seven-day 155-mile stage run in the Gobi Desert. She did not do this as part of her normal work routine but solely as a volunteer. But upon completion of the grueling foot race, her potential to grow the program was seen by her supervisors and she was offered an ambassadorship. Soon she found herself on the Board of Directors with Runwell. Now she helps guide the ship which once threw her a life preserver.

Addiction is tragic but recovery is more powerful. Recently, Pam attended the wedding of her youngest daughter. As a wedding present she and he husband were given wine goblets to commemorate the occasion. Pam sees this as a symbolic, if not rather accidental, gesture. A few years ago she might not have made it out of the reception before breaking out the goblet and filling it with wine. Today she uses the same fervor with which she threw alcohol in her throat to help others break free and move forward with their lives. She knows how fleeting life can be.

If her own addiction was not enough of a reminder of how quickly one's life can change, Pam need only look to that iconic Boston Marathon. She finally decided to run the race that helped kick start her new world in 2009. She returned a few more times until she almost became a statistic in 2013. Pam, like thousands of other runners at the Boston Marathon and millions nationwide could have never expected the finish line to be a place of anything other than triumph and relief. Yet, when bombs ripped through the crowd of runners, just minutes after she passed by the very spot where they lie, the Boston Marathon took on a whole new meaning for virtually everyone. Pam had to wait hours to get even a text through to her loved ones, while they hoped and prayed she was uninjured. She realized how easily those calls could have gone, unheard by herself, waiting to be returned if any of her DUIs had gone the wrong way.

She mentions how she wore a Boston Marathon jacket for a week after the bombing almost in a silent showing of solidarity. By doing so, and taking it to expos at many different races this jacket is now filled with the signatures of those like Frank Shorter, Bart Yasso, Bill Rodgers, and Meb Keflezghi. These athletes who inspire her are all people she would have never met if she had continued down the destructive path she had trotted on for years. Now, instead her path is filled with trees and trails and balloon-laced finish lines.

That's a fairly decent trade-off.

3

Meagan Nedlo

There are many ways to start your marathon career. Without a doubt, one of the worst would be by not even getting to the finish line of your first two marathons. Then again, it is hard to argue with the means when the end result has you participating in the Olympic Trials not too long after.

Meagan Nedlo took a rather circuitous route to one of the most illustrious running stages. In 7th grade track she was undefeated in the unlikely combo of 100-meter hurdles and the mile. This led to her decision as a freshman to join the track and cross-country teams. There were no groundbreaking times or Runner's World cover stories but on those teams in her small town of Pittsburg, TX, she did just fine, thank you very much. By the time her high school career ended she was a solidly self-described "mediocre" 12-minute two-miler. While this is a time many would love to have, it is also good to keep it in perspective that this type of speed means the phone wasn't ringing off the hook with scholarship offers. This hard bothered Meagan. She figured her competitive running career was more or less over, just like it is for thousands of those who like to run across the nation come every graduation.

Enrolling at Texas Christian University in Dallas, she still ran frequently and exercised consistently. There was no structured training to her life or daily schedule of running. However, she was sure to make it a point not to let her running fitness go stale. Also, while there did not necessarily seem to be much in store for her in the elite running world, she did not let it get out of her sights. After graduation, she began working in the running industry, first for Mizuno and then for Brooks. She found herself constantly surrounded by other people who loved running just as much as she did. Meagan hardly needed any needling with regard to loving the sport of running. But now, since she was constantly around those who simply loved to run, it was making it impossible not to catch the bug herself. Her dabbling was now over and she decided to get more serious with her training.

Slowly Meagan began to get take to her workouts with more purpose. She started competing in local races. Her times showed signs of hidden talent or at least a good lung capacity. With an 18:45 5k time and somewhere in the neighborhood of thirty-nine minutes for a 10k she knew that perhaps she had left some stones unturned. She was happy to continue to push the envelope in the shorter distances but as anyone in the running world knows, the most anyone wants to talk about is whether or not you have done a marathon. So, Meagan thought about giving it a go. Her friend Jordan, one heck of a runner in his own right, suggested she speak to his friend and former college teammate, Jeff Gaudette, as a coach. Jeff just so happened to be the assistant coach for track and field as well as cross-country at Queens University in Charlotte, NC. This will soon come into play. Pay attention.

Jeff coached Meagan remotely through emailed workouts. He never once had the opportunity to be on-hand for Meagan while she pushed herself solo through tough days and even tougher days. However, at some point in her training Jeff became convinced of her potential to do more. Upon doing some research into the abyss that is the NCAA regulations, he concluded Meagan still had collegiate eligibility. At that point he took it upon himself to call Meagan up and say:

"How would you like to quit your job, move to Charlotte and run for Queens while getting your master's degree?"

Apparently, she thought about it as long as a goldfishes' memory and jumped at the chance. And that's the story as to how Meagan began her first collegiate track season at the ripe old age of 26.

In her short time competing at the collegiate level (just two season of track and one of cross country was all she was eligible for), Meagan showed her coach he had guessed correctly. She earned three All-American honors during her second track season at Queens in 2010 (5000 meter indoors, 5000 and 10,000 outdoors). Her teammate Tanya Zeferjahn and she then placed 5th as a team at Outdoor Nationals. This finish just happened to be the highest NCAA finish of any sports team in Queens' school history. As for those nice, but just nice times in her 5k and 10k? Well, they were destroyed and lowered to 16:35 and 34:35, respectively. Not only was running this fast beyond what most could expect for a late-20s frosh, it was leaps and bounds above what Meagan ever believed she'd be capable of doing.

When you have this sort of talent, you will inevitably find yourself at the starting line of a marathon no matter how much you like running the short stuff. Right outside of the US Marine Corps War Memorial (sometimes referred to as the Iwo Jima Memorial) is where Meagan decided to break through that barrier in October of 2008 at the famed Marine Corps Marathon. It surprised her that it actually took this long to get here. Her thought process from high school on was that running marathons is what runners who weren't signed to shoe contract did. If you were an adult, and you didn't run in college, you probably just ran in marathons. Now, she was finally joining their ranks. She was going to become a marathon runner.

Unfortunately, while she started the race, she didn't finish it. She had to drop out at mile 18. Stopping wasn't something that had been on her agenda when she started but it became a part of her reality now. While she knew it was the right choice it was not the one she wanted to make. Her first attempt at taking on 26.22 miles was a failure.

Her next marathon would be different, though. Roughly half a year after she finished her eligibility at Queens, her training began anew. She picked the Houston Marathon in 2011 as a goal race for several different reasons. First, it's a fast course. Second, she knew that's where the Olympic trials were going to be the next year. She had a feeling in her gut she could make those trials and running the course in advance would be greatly helpful. Finally, being from Texas, her family could come to cheer her on without having to make a cross-country flight. In her mind, everything would be perfect. This was the best opportunity for her to run a 2:44 or maybe a 2:45. Her workouts had not been up to what she knew she could do but when are they ever, really? She figured she had the mental toughness, the fresh legs and the training to get her through. Then she got to the race.

Texas weather is notoriously mercurial. Even though Houston's marathon weather is traditionally cold, her day broke warm and muggy. By the halfway point, she could tell that it just wasn't going to be her race. Again. Her half split was right on target to get what she needed but by mile 17 she was on the sidelines.

There was no spinning this positively. Meagan was crushed. Her parents were there to support her. Friends running the US Half Marathon Championships the day before had lined the course to cheer her on. Everyone on Facebook knew this was going to be her big day. But it all came floundering down nine miles from the actual finish. She didn't have a bad time or miss her goal. She got the dreaded. She was now 0-2 for even getting to the finish line of a marathon. Her doubts grew greatly about whether she was the type of runner she had come to think she might be.

Just two weeks later, Meagan found herself working the expo at the Mercedes Marathon in Birmingham, AL. There had been no plan to run a race here of any distance, let alone the marathon. Instead, she had come to the race to stand for two straight days on hard expos floors. Both authors have done this and tried running a race the next day. Lt's just say it is about the most exhausting thing you can do. But for some reason, Meagan decided she might as well give the marathon one more go. Heck, she was here, right?

She ate a random non-specific dinner at a friend's house. She slept on a couch. There were no special bottles placed out for her as an elite runner. She received no special treatment other than her friend simply dropping her off at the start. No one was on the course to cheer for her. No one on social media even knew she was running. This race was done simply to see if she really should hang it up and stick to the short races. Her time goals were barely existent. She just wanted to finish. If she failed, no one even needed to know she ran. The last thing she wanted to do was come back to a myriad of condolences from well-meaning friends asking her to more or less re-live her failure a thousand times over.

On a course that was far more challenging than that of the Houston Marathon, Meagan did not fold. The weather cooperated; she hit on all cylinders, and ran her heart out. Her weary expo legs carried her to a stellar time of 2:45:00 on the nose. Her first completed marathon ever was a full minute under the Women's "B" Olympic Trials qualifying standard. She grabbed the 3rd women overall in the entire race. Meagan finally had some redemption.

A few months later, thoughts of a potential fall marathon to prove her run at Birmingham was not a fluke, fell by the wayside. The Mercedes Marathon had simply taken too much out of her. She had always respected the distance but know she fully understood what it took to run this hard for this long. It took so much from not only her body but her mind and soul as well. So instead of possibly floundering in another marathon attempt, she went with shorter races to work on her leg speed and turnover.

Right when she was hitting her stride a promotion in her shoe company of Karhu had her leaving her nest of fast friends in North Carolina woods. She found herself moving north to the greater Boston area, where cold winters and harsh weather awaited. Moreover, the move happened right when the most important part of her training for the Olympic Trials was underway.

Somehow, amidst all the turmoil off life, Meagan made it work. She entered the Olympic Trials fit and ready for a new personal best. In addition, the pressure was gone. One does not get to the trials unless they are, in any one's definition "fast". But there is "fast" and there is *fast*. Meagan was aware she was not the one which requires italics in the written word. While she would be running as hard as she could, she knew there was a completely different race going on at the front. This race was a battle amongst just a handful in which she need not concern herself. All she had to do was run her own pace and let the cards fall where they may.

Seeded close to 150th out of all the runners, Meagan was simply happy to be on the starting line. She was back in her home state with weather much more to her liking that the year before. Her fans and friends were on-hand but they were secondary to her race. Meagan simply had to run the effort she knew she was capable of doing. The rest would be decided by things out of her control. Well, a four- minute PR, a 2:41 finish and a top 50 overall place is what this day netted her.

What makes Meagan's story rather unique is something a few runners who work in the industry can relate to: being a runner and working in the running world is often horrible for your running. Running jobs are rarely desk jobs. These jobs have you on your feet constantly at expos and trade shows. Long hours of talking and eating bad food, and being at the beck and call of hundreds of potential customers are what await you. Squatting to tie shoes, sizing up people, doing presentations. Getting a run in is usually one of the hardest things a runner can actually do. Now imagine all of that when you are trying to be one of the fastest fifty women in the entire country. Not exactly a "dream job" so to speak, now is it?

But that is the story of life. Few things go even remotely close to perfect. Meagan has since lowered her marathon PR to 2:39:02. She always seems right on that minute mark just missing the next big milestone. Going u der 2:39 would have secured her the "A" standard for the US Women's Trials. Yet she knows she has the talent and the drive to go faster. She has done all of this in the most unconventional of ways. A late bloomer who works full-time and more or less treats running as a hobby. A hobby that she works exceedingly hard at while excelling under difficult circumstances. She doesn't have a cushy job or two-a- day workouts filled with nothing other than naps and massages and eating. That lifestyle is for the very lucky few. Meagan is not one of them.

However, her story is one that inspires us all. A great deal of you reading this book are late bloomers when it comes to the running world. You got here by your own story but can easily relate to the ups and downs Meagan has experienced. She has learned that limiting oneself is the biggest hurdle. If you think the fastest you have already run is the fastest you will ever run, then you have already dug your own grave. No one can hurdle walls that are planted in their own mind.

Meagan believes she can run a 2:35 or faster in the marathon. Even as she has passed over the 30-year-old barrier she has shown age is not a deciding factor in where you go. Nor does being competitive mean you can't still care about your friends. Most notably, one of the training partners Meagan ran with so religiously in North Carolina with, Caitlin, was running step by step with her in a race aptly titled Heart and Sole Women's 5 miler. A race comprised solely of those with the XY chromosomes, the race was a celebration of women's running. The ending celebrated it even more.

About halfway through the race, Meagan and Caitlin decided that if they were close at the finish, they would honor the camaraderie of women runners by running hard but finishing together. So when the finish line appeared the two women grabbed hands and in a show of solidarity, tied for first place. They split the prize money, the overall award but kept their friendship united. It inspired floods of questions and media opportunity but for Meagan it was giving back a little to one of the women who had helped get her to the finish line in the first place.

Running often rewards those who thank it for what is has given them. Meagan just started getting rewarded a little later than most.

4

Kris Graci

The reason why we empathize with stories of people who have lost loved ones is because we have all walked that road. Unlike trying to understand what it is like to lose a limb or have your eyesight taken, we do not need to use our imagination. We have all been on the other end of that phone call when we suddenly learn someone we cared about was simply no longer with us. Regardless of whether it was a surprise or a long time in the making, we understand having the wind knocked out of us. For Kris Graci, getting knocked down seemed to be the wake-up call every single day for the span of a year and a half. She took the one-two punch on the chin, answered the bell and got pummeled some more.

In just 18 months, Kris had to deal with the death of her husband, her mother, her grandmother, her uncle and a close personal family friend. For good measure, we might as well mention her family dog died as did her cat. One minute each and every one of them was in her life; the next minute, they were gone forever.

Few things prepare us for the death of a family member. When a slew of them come in quick succession, there truly is no handbook that will make things any easier. For Kris, the usual people she would turn to for solace or understanding were the very ones she was losing to mortality. She was at an absolute loss as to how to handle each successive death. So, she tried baking.

Food became, as it does for so many, a crutch on which a deeply saddened person can depend. Given the immense depth of the sadness for Kris, the baking was equally immense. Unfortunately, even though she was giving much of the food away, a far larger portion that she needed was finding its way to her own mouth. Her weight ballooned.

Kris wasn't a runner. She wasn't a cyclist. Walks to the park were not in her vocabulary. Even the small exercise she would get with her dog was taken away from her. Physical activity was simply not part of her life. In fact, the most rigorous things she did on a daily basis was chewing or knitting. She got very good at both.

With her skills in knitting she took people under her wing. She started teaching others her craft. People would come to her door asking for scarves or afghan blankets or other knitted items. Kris loved that she could make other people happy. It went a great deal to helping her forget about her own unhappiness. Her darning became damn good. However, the problem with even being a world-class knitter is, you are burning, at most, about seven calories per hour. (There is no data out there on how many calories knitting burns but this is probably pretty darn close.)

The weight she was putting on was not a surprise to Kris. However, she used the extra weight as a metaphoric shield. This buffer protected her from the uppercuts and body blows of her recent losses. She understood why it was called comfort food and she needed a great deal of comfort. One day, however, she knew she had to make a change. It dawned upon her that if she kept up grieving in this fashion, soon others would be grieving for her. So she decided to deal with a grief in a different way. Kris decided to go to the gym.

Her main idea was to at least spend time away from the home and more specifically the kitchen. Even if she wasn't doing any exercise, at least she wouldn't be baking foods to eat. She hired a personal trainer to start her along. She knew she couldn't exercise outside, in plain sight. The last thing she wanted to do was to be seen outside running, especially in the shape she was in. So she got on the treadmill and hated every single solitary step.

Eventually, she realized the hatred was not of running but of why she was even in the gym in the first place. While he wouldn't be posing for the cover of an ESPN Bodies Issue anytime soon, prior to all the turmoil in her life, she certainly wasn't obese. The rough hand she had been dealt had facilitated her gaining the weight. Instead of shielding her when she thought how out of shape she was, it took her back to the genesis of the weight gain. Losing the pounds would go a long way to losing the constant reminders of how suddenly alone she felt.

She grabbed a friend, walked into the popular Running Room store near her home in Canada and joined a couch to 5k program. She decided to make chewing miles her new habit.

When you speak with Kris about this first 5k she ran you feel like you are almost at the finish line with her. She waxes poetic, almost reverentially, about those final few steps. She paints a picture which catches you and makes you smile right along with her. The time on the clock is irrelevant. Her overall place meant nothing. The only thing that matters was that finish line was her starting line to the rest of her healthy life. But it would still be a struggle.

Even while she was chasing further and further distances, the reality was that Kris was running from reality. She had gotten over the initial grief of having lost so many loved ones but now the longer-term realities start to set in. Kris has two daughters and one is getting married soon. Knowing that her husband will not be there with her to help celebrate this momentous occasion is crushing. Yet, she does what she can to strengthen her resolve.

She is spending time leading up to that day looking for, in her words, that one dress which says, "YES! You found me." This same dress will spark years of memories and smiles even while it reminds her of who will never see it. Kris smiles and is happy for her daughter but at the same time can't help but tear up inside. The man who raised her daughter won't be there to give her away. She never planned on having to be this strong. She doesn't know exactly how she should react. Should she hide her emotions? Should she let them flow? The questions are many and the answers are few. But the emotions are there and they are raw.

Kris will still come home from a race and have the instinct to go and show her husband the medal before remembering he is not there to see it. Sometimes she breaks down and cries. Other times she simply stares into space, wishing he were there to see what she has done. Reality smacks her and reminds her she is now a widow. Fortunately, her family is all about living.

Both her daughters are in the health care profession. One actually has taken on the half-marathon distance. Ironically, she did so before Kris started running and claims she will never run another again. But you can tell Kris would love few things more than to toe the line of a race with her children. She would love to share with them the cathartic release of putting one foot in front of the other. In fact, her soon to be son-in-law took part in the Round the Bay 30k in Canada, the oldest race in North America. As he was a bit faster than Kris, they did not see much of each other during the race. However, when she crossed the line, he was there waiting to envelope her in a hug.

Kris still indulges in the occasional "turtle blizzard chocolate dipped waffle cone" but the days of constant eating are behind her. Her circle of friends now includes runners, cyclists and adventure athletes. Races are her version of the psychiatrist's couch. She uses races to deal with the losses she can never forget. With no husband and no mother to be able to share her experiences with she has instead turned to her daughters and the nameless masses. The runners around her for a few hours on race day have become her family. Kris, like all of us, looks to the running community to be a surrogate family. In some ways, Kris is every single one of us.

If this was the end of the story, we could all pretend everything will be perfectly fine for Kris. But her story goes deeper. You see, about two months prior to her husbands' death, Kris was in a car accident. Because of the litany of horrible things that happened in her life soon thereafter, her own accident was pushed to page two. In fact, Kris never even went to the hospital.

Fast-forward two years and a discovery was made. Dizziness and headaches, which were originally thought to be a by-product of the anti-depressants she was taking to cope with grief, were found to have another cause. The car accident had given Kris not only a concussion but also cerebral damage. She now has extremely bad short-term memory. The knitting she used to love has all but disappeared from her life. She lacks the skills and concentration to complete the task. She often looks longingly at the objects she once crafted. The envy of the neighborhood, they are now another reminder of things that once existed.

Kris wishes she could knit again. But she doesn't wallow in self-pity. Even though she occasionally forgets which races she has even run, she knows having fun in each one is the most important thing. Furthermore, as have been proven many times by various people worldwide, running helps with cognition. Kris knows running is helping to combat her memory loss. She is hoping continuing to do so will help her win this battle as well. It already removed the pounds. Now maybe it will add the memories. Regardless, for the time she is running, life has clarity and serenity.

Kris could look at her story as one of woe. She could easily have taken what has been handed to her and made it a crutch. Excuses would actually be reasons and no one could really blame her. Instead, almost miraculously, she has taken this myriad of negatives and turned them into positives. She is happy with what she has. While she could have rolled over and accepted that life was perfectly happy kicking her when she was down, she took the harder route. She stood up even when it was literally difficult to do so. She turned her life around. She refused to be a victim. With each finish line she crosses she proves she is a fighter. But she is a lover too.

In fact, if you want a hug, it is really simple. Just find out Kris' running schedule and position yourself on the route. Chances are better than average she will go out of her way to make sure you get one.

5

Heather Alvarado

On the surface, Heather Alvarado has a story similar to many of today's runners. Not much of a runner growing up, she developed a case of what I like to call "Adult Onset Running". She discovered what running did for her both mentally and physically and now cannot imagine her world existing without it.

Below the surface, there is a much more involved story. Heather's mother, Linda, made history in 1992 when she became the first Latino owner of a Major League Baseball team, male or female. Helming the Colorado Rockies was just one of the many illustrious firsts for Linda Alvarado. Growing up in a poor family of six in New Mexico, her achievements have been hard to top. As such, you can imagine being the offspring of such a successful person brings with it a modicum of expectations. This can be both good and bad.

Heather mentions how growing up with such a groundbreaking person as her mom was rather intimidating. At the same time, while everyone saw a pioneer, she simply saw her mom telling her it was time to go to bed or to eat her vegetables. Seeing how even the most successful of people are just, in fact, people really instilled a sense of evenness in her life. She appreciated the work ethic her mother had and tried to emulate her strength. There would be many times she would need it later in life.

In junior high, a group of friends whom Heather considered her best friends all decided they wished to join the cheerleading team. Heather felt she would rather be playing sports than cheering others on to victory. She expected these friends to support her decision. However, she found that rather than see what she wanted to do as simply an independent person setting off on her own path, they instead ostracized her. She was crushed.

She knows looking back she made the right decision. She had to go her own way. Following others down a path that wasn't for her would have made her one of the sheep. An adult woman can look back and see how this was the correct choice. A teenage girl, who just lost what she thought was her support group, is, however a different story. As junior high bled into high school, not much changed with regards to Heather seeking out her own life choices. She thinks if she had been a runner back then, life would have been a great deal easier.

She graduated from high school in Colorado and was pushed by her mother to chase after what she felt were her passions. For Heather, who now considered herself part punk rocker and part artist, film and art school beckoned. For her there was no better place than New York City to take on those challenges.

While in New York, the idea of running never entered her mind. She was a little brooding and a bit aloof. Getting up at the crack of dawn to run for fifteen miles was simply absurd. She had heard of the New York City Marathon just like everyone else but never thought about participating in anything of its ilk. Running was for people who had leisure time to spare. They had problems that they needed to escape from and running was their way to do so. She was far too busy with her studies and her craft to do something so frivolous. The dalliances of others, short shorts and all, was not for her.

She spent a brief period of time in Oxford, England. Here, interestingly enough was where she would ride her bike by the home of the writer and poet C. S. Lewis almost every day. The author known by many for his *Chronicles of Narnia* saga also has a quote with which many runners can identify.

"If one could run without getting tired, I don't think one would often want to do anything else."

At the time, however, this was not Heather. Today, she cannot imagine ever having a persona not shaped by these exact words.

Heather got married while she lived in New York City but soon thereafter moved back to Colorado. Before leaving, a series of incidents led to Heather seeking some medical attention wherein she learned she was bipolar. But the diagnosis did little to quell the irrational fears or the mood swings. The highs were off the chart and the lows subterranean. The medication she was given did little to help so, like so many, she turned to self-medicating. Cocaine became her drug of choice.

Back in Colorado, she continued to use cocaine and was "getting by" in her own words. Her husband, however, was unhappy and wanted to move to Los Angeles to be a writer. Heather promised they would move but it is hard to put money in the bank when it is instead going up your nose. Heather admits she was a skillful liar and no one knew the problem she had. Moreover, they didn't know her marriage was failing.

One day her husband packed a suitcase and left. He texted from a local bar saying he wanted a divorce with nary a phone call. Heather had a nervous breakdown. She quit her job, holed herself in her apartment and wouldn't speak to anyone. After a period of time, her brother-in-law finally cracked her entryway and saw the emotional and physical wreckage inside. Heather knew she needed help.

She checked herself into a rehab clinic, expecting to stay for one month. She was there for three times that length. Then another three-month stay followed in Hollywood. After that, another three months in Malibu. Finally, after nine total months of living clean, she gathered the strength to move back to her family in Colorado.

Her therapist who she saw quite frequently suggested she take her obvious addictive personality and turn it into a new hobby. Perhaps she could take up painting or work on her art again. Maybe, as others found it successful in helping them deal, she could try running. Heather thought it might work for her.

For two years, Heather never entered a race. Running was not a means to an end with regards to training for a distance. The mere act of ambulation meant she was in control. Lacing up her shoes was a powerful thing. Getting home and kicking those shoes off after a run was an achievement. Her first three-miler was cause for celebration. When she toppled a double-digit run you would have thought her mother's team had won the World Series she was so excited. Each time she pushed further and strained at what she thought was possible, she took herself further away from the drugs, the bad marriage and her own bad habits.

She had been dating a man who she met at one of her AA meeting. A former heroin user he was very supportive of her running even though he himself wasn't a runner. For two years they were a healthy couple. Unfortunately, her boyfriend's resolve was not the same as Heather's. She soon noticed money missing and his mood changing. He was stealing from her to feed his habit. Heather, herself on the giving end of the lies she was now receiving saw the telltale signs. But she was powerless to help.

One night she watched a little television and went to bed. When she woke up the next morning, the house smelled of gas. She tried to track down the source and followed her nose to the garage. Here she found her boyfriend. He had gone in the car, shot of up a ton of heroin and died. Heather found both his suicide note and his body. She crumbled.

Needless to say, her life was turned upside down again. She felt the downward spiral coming but did not know how to stop it. Slumping around for a few months she found her answer in the note her boyfriend had penned to her. "Please never give up running."

Fortunately for Heather, when she needed the running scene the most, the running scene was really getting into Colorado. She joined running groups in her area and grew up right along with them. She was now in her mid-30s and ready to take on actual racing. She needed something to help lift this painful fog from her life. Soon she was taking on the entire smorgasbord of events the scene in Colorado could offer.

Running became integral in how she saw herself. In fact, she dreams of owning a running store someday. In the meantime she has thrown herself headlong into programs which offer others outlets she did not have. At the top of her list is Girls on the Run (GOTR), a program that empowers young girls to know their own value by staying active and fit. For four years, Heather has been a coach for GOTR, where she emphasizes the strength one can have by keeping both their mind and body strong.

In addition, Heather has taken her own running to a level she could have never thought possible. Her age group trophies might not be the envy of the elite but they more than fill the space she could have ever imagined needing growing up. But where she finds the most value is in continuing to help others. She has raised money for countless charities through running, and even gone so far as to assist visually impaired runners in races.

As running came to her so much later in life, she feels she was robbed of some opportunities to enjoy it to its fullest when she was younger. While she loves any activity which gets people running, the niche races today where people don't seem to be out there to give their best irk her a little bit. Having seen how easily life can be snubbed out, not giving your all in what you do seem like a waste to her. She does not care so much what your time is as much as you gave all you had when you got to the starting line.

The girl who lost friends and went down a dark path because of not wanting to be a cheerleader now finds so much pleasure in doing just that. For Heather, the only thing better than pushing as hard as she can to achieve what she knows is within her power is watching her friends do the same thing. And while she might not have pom-poms there won't be anyone at the finish screaming more loudly than she.

6

Michelle Walker

We have reached a time in our society where every single person thinks they are busy. Of course, being busy is relative. In addition, being busy does not automatically mean you are being productive. Michelle Walker, however, is definitely both.

Known affectionately as Mom O'Six because she collects raccoon figurines (We are kidding; she has six kids. Just making sure you are reading closely), Michelle makes the absolute most out of the twenty-four hours each day brings.

Catching up with Michelle is the hardest part. In the fall of 2014, Michelle was readying herself for one of her many marathons, this time taking place in Africa. It would be her 90th lifetime marathon. Yet in spite of this incredible achievement, she will be almost as nervous when she goes to the start of this race as she was when she toed the line of her first marathon. She knows that this distance will challenge her every time. There are always factors out of her control that makes each race unique. Some days it is the weather, others the course provides the challenge and sometimes, well, it is just mind games she tries to ignore which provide the challenge.

However, what makes Michelle different from many multiple marathon finishers is her desire to improve her marathon race times as often as possible. She has gradually reduced her time from the 4:10 range to her latest personal record personal record of 3:29. This fastest time was achieved at the 2013 Tucson Marathon, one known to give a little to runners in the way of downhill but take a great deal back from the pounding the quads take on those same hills. But Michelle excels at taking what is given to her and making it work.

Since her teenage years, exercise has been part of her daily routine. She does not necessarily see it as a chore as much as something she must do. Like brushing her teeth or eating, exercise is simply a necessity. Feeling we are only given one body, Michelle feels the responsibility of keeping hers in peak physical condition falls squarely on her shoulders. She also knows that life intervenes. In other words, there are times when reasons will exist where her running might have to take a backseat. But she never tries to make excuses for being fit. Instead, she makes time.

When one has a family, which includes six children ranging in ages from 19 to 5, there is no set schedule. Fortunately, one of her children is already navigated the busy Walker household and is in college. So while one of her offspring might not need the same level of care as the others, the fact Michelle has done what she has while making sure her son succeeded in school and life, is amazing in itself. But with five other children under her roof, fitting her runs into her family's schedule often means setting her alarm for 5 a.m. Maybe earlier.

If her lifestyle simply meant she had to wake up early to grab a run before her children woke, those early mornings wouldn't mean much. However in order to travel the way she does, which is often for such a brief stay that she barely needs to fill the gas tank in the rental car, it also entails planning ahead and arranging childcare. Obviously, races away from home require intricate planning but given the varying schedules of so many children, even the long runs when she is simply stepping foot outside her door require for her to plan a week (or more) in advance. Kids; commitments must be met with children getting rides to where they need to go, all over town to multiple different schools, functions, sports, etc.

Michelle knows she is fortunate. Not every mother has the stability of her family or the ability to make ends meet as she does. She knows she is lucky she is to have the loving support of family. Without them, completing a marathon in each of the 50 states would have been impossible. Yet that is what Michelle has done.

While her parents did not live right next door, a quick two hour drive has them being able to spend time with their grandchildren on the occasions where Michelle must hit the road. Many times, Michelle will take her children with her on a road trip, eschewing the closer airports to her home to drop them off at her parents' house, which is closer to another airport. There is some time she does miss in her family's life but her children get to see their grandparents more often and longer than many families who are much more sedentary.

Many of the trips she takes, her children come with her. Her family calls these excursions "runcations". While Michelle is busting her hump slogging through another 26.2 miles, her family's lives are enriched by the places they go.

Her family has not grown in the traditional sense (there appears to me no need for the moniker to change to Mom o'7 anytime soon) but because of running, many more people are in her life than would not have been. The Loneliness of the Long Distance Runner was a short story made popular by Alan Sillitoe and for a while to those outsiders who never logged a mile, it characterized runners. Loners. Out on a run in the wee hours of the morning or night. On a country run in a blizzard. A solo figure against the elements. For a time, that description was rather true. But today that is different. Running is no longer a fringe sport populated by the skinny few running 100 mile weeks wearing socks as gloves in cotton sweatshirts. Now, as a sport of the masses it encompasses all walks of life. As such, it allows more and more people to become greater friends with those they may have never met otherwise. For Michelle, it means her family has grown.

She was once under the impression held by many that running is a solitary activity. She has found in the past seven years she could not have been more wrong. For Michelle, the biggest reward she has received has nothing to do with trophies or shiny finisher medals. Rather, the friendships she has made are the shiny baubles she cherishes most. Relationships have been formed and strengthened locally, nationally, and even internationally through running. While other friendships may tarnish and fade her running friends seem to be the ones who will be there for life. Runners know about hard times. They know about long periods where things do not go right. More than just about anyone else, runners seem to be perfectly suited for friendship, especially the kind separated by distance and time.

For Michelle, the camaraderie she has stumbled upon in the running world has changed her life. The support and enjoyment she feels pouring in from her running friends has made her a much happier person. This happiness spills over into her family life, making her a better mom and wife.

Included in what running has given her are the amazing places and sights her racing has taken her. She has been to every state in the union. The Caribbean islands of the Bahamas and Puerto Rico are on her crossed-off list. From Chile to Spain and from Zimbabwe to Tokyo, Michelle has seen the world 26.2 miles at a time. Did I forget to mention Antarctica?

In fact, not only did she complete a marathon in Antarctica, she did so a day after completing another marathon in Chile. The races were not intentionally scheduled to be that close together. On an excursion to Antarctica, the marathon on the frozen continent continued to get delayed because of nasty weather. Michelle and others stewed in Chile as days went by. Given the weather, it appeared as if the race in Antarctica would never happen. So, the runners decided to go ahead with the originally schedule time for the marathon in Chile, which was supposed to be after the one in Antarctica. You have to roll with the punches sometimes.

Upon finishing the marathon, the tour group told the runners the weather had broken. Michelle, standing sweaty in her running clothes was basically informed it was now or never to get on the creaky watery vessel which would take them to the Great White South. When the Russian freighter says it is time to go, well it is usually not the tourists who get to say nyet. On board Michelle and her group went, jamming clothing they would need for the next day in bags with them. All the careful planning and relaxing and refueling went out the window. Less than a day later she was dancing amongst penguins.

Her marathon to the Victoria Falls Marathon in Zimbabwe was a little less hectic but jammed with as much as one possibly should when they are still tackling 26.2 miles of running. The untamed wildness won Michelle over and quickly became her favorite trip yet. While in the area, she and her family were able to visit three other African countries, fully experiencing the wildlife, beauty, and hospitality of the region. Then she squeezed out a marathon and came home. Just another weekend for the Walkers.

Running is not just a vacation for Michelle. It is her oxygen mask. It's the white noise that she gets to listen to around the jammed-packed reality of her life. She loves being a mother of six but she loves still simply being Michelle. Running is often the only time she can carve out of the day where she can organize her thoughts. It is during this time where she really can think about the needs of her children. Who needs to go where? Which child would benefit from a little extra care or love that week? How she can make sure that each new trip enriches the children even more?

Let's face it, no matter how good your children are, if there are six of them, you sometimes need a break. Not only does running serve as her preferred method of physical fitness, it is her number one stress reliever. Running brings her back to where she can handle the rigors of being a mom and a wife and an event organizer for a bunch of very need clients. Children can often be seen as uncompromising CEOs.

But moreover her children have seen what a transition can come from being around a mother who exercises. The physical and mental benefits of not just running, but of exercise in general, are not lost on these children. Michelle has made it a priority to model and talk to them about the importance of an exercise routine. She is starting to reap the benefits of this on-hand lesson plan. Most of her children have competed in some races of some distance. Her oldest son ran cross-country in high school and now her oldest daughter has competed in races ranging up to 10 miles. When they cross the finish line it is a victory for Michelle almost as much as it is for them.

But do not think she is living her life through her children. She is living her life through herself, which makes her children wish to do the same thing. There is no pressure to compete. No pressure to run. The only pressure comes from a mother who wishes to make sure her children know the value of an honest sweat.

She hopes to model a healthy lifestyle for her children but also is putting into action goal setting behavior through marathon running. Her kids are interested in the progress she makes towards her running goals. Unlike many kids who can be embarrassed by their parents, her children are proud that their mom accomplished a monumental goal of completing a marathon in each state. The fact she is also trying to run a 26.2 miler on every continent enthralls them even more. While the younger ones still think the only reason someone would be going to this amount of effort would be to set a world record, Michelle knows she is not doing this for a gold medal or a piece of paper certifying her as a Guinness record holder. She is doing it because it is now part of her.

She is not the same person she was before she started marathoning. She is more fulfilled. She has a renewed zest for life and more self-confidence. Her organization skills are better and she can tend to the needs of my family more easily now.

It is easy to find reasons why some of us can do the things we do and others cannot. Some might not have the same supportive family as Michelle. Some might not have the means to hire a babysitter if they don't have the family for help. Others might not have children but have responsibilities, which make it difficult to do the things they would really wish to do. But with life there is sacrifice. None of us really get to do all the things we want to do. We have to pick and choose.

At the beginning of this chapter, the busy nature of our culture was touched upon. The reason we did so here while talking with Michelle is we know very few people who have more on their plate. Yet Michelle wanted to accomplish something, so she is working to make it happen. She sacrifices sleep so she can get in her runs before her motherly duties begin. She flies crazy schedules in order to spend as little as time as possible away from her family. And, when possible, she takes the whole brood with her. Her children are learning about hard-work and sacrifice while also getting a first-hand view of the world as it changes. They see a woman who could easily say "Hey, being a mom of six kids who are healthy and happy and doing well in their respective plays, sports, school, etc. is more than enough of an achievement. I don't need to do anything else!"

She doesn't need to, she wants to. So she does.

7

Myla Johnson

Myla Johnson has cheated death, survived the loss of loved ones in horrific ways and done so through the sometimes waning support of those closest to her. The strength and resolve necessary to get through such trying emotional challenges can be seen in Myla throughout her life. It may also be able to be traced back to a non-existent track team.

Myla has always liked to run. She enjoyed the wind on her face and the sound it made whistling by her ears. She felt it gave her a freedom unsurpassed by any other means of locomotion. When she was just twelve she laced up her running shoes knowing when she started 7th grade she would try out for the girls track team. The only problem with that plan was in small Clay City, Indiana; there was no girls' team.

We often make fun of the way children ask questions. Comedian Louis C.K. has a legendary comedy sketch about how there is not answer to a child's question of "why?" They always have another "why?" in the barrel to fire at you. But something must be said for the way children solve problems.

There is a matter-of-factness amongst them that is missing in adults. In this particular instance, when Myla heard there was no girls' team, she looked around and saw a team with boys. Why shouldn't she simply join the team with boys? So she did.

Unfortunately, although she made the team, a slight uproar followed. There are a variety of sports in small towns that are mixed gender. As such, wondering if the genders are fairly matched in order to keep the children safe is an intelligent thing. Ironically, however, at young ages, it is usually the girls who are taller or faster or stronger than the majority of the boys. In addition, with the sport of running there is no difficult question as to whether an athlete is good enough or not to make the team. There are no intangibles to ascertain or worries over different body types between the sexes. With running, you simply run the distance and look at the clock. Who was fastest? What was the next person in line? Who was last? It is all pretty straightforward. At least it should be.

In the end, despite her obvious talent level, at least compared to her peers, Myla was not allowed to join the boy's team. Fortunately, her attempt to show how easily girls could run with the boys opened some eyes in the community. While she was not allowed to become a member of her 7th grade boy's track team, she did become part of the inaugural girls team. Score one for perseverance and the energy and wisdom of youth.

But succeeding against obstacles was nothing new for this tomboy. Myla was used to taking on challenges headfirst. She knows often the fights she would choose would be the ones who hit back. Yet she was ready for them. It often seems the people who are made of the toughest stuff, the ones with the intestinal fortitude, are the ones the fates like to challenge the most.

The team in which Myla helped create was a jumping off point. It was the building block of a refuge would retreat to many times in her life. Running would constantly become the place where she could go and know its safety and warmth. The familiarity of putting on shoes and getting in a good run would be what she needed to get through tough times. As a child, however, she was simply happy to have been named the most valuable long distance runner. The road ahead, however, would test that endurance.

Myla enrolled at East Tennessee State University. Luckily, she did not have to fight for the creation of any teams in Johnson City, Tennessee. She also didn't necessarily have the talent to be part of those times, either. Regardless, she was still running for fitness and for fun. It was what she knew best. Then life decided to test her resolve. Her boyfriend back home, Jack, died in a car accident. Myla's life was thrown into upheaval.

She lost all her appetite. She wasn't able to sleep. Classes were becoming an afterthought as she walked through life in a semi-comatose state. The pain and grief of having someone she cared about so much taken away from her so violently made everything else secondary. Soon she found herself in a full-blown case of anorexia nervosa.

The strong runner with the smallish frame of 5'4" who had imposed her will on a school district to start a track team to accommodate her (and other girl's) wishes was now being laid to waste by an eating disorder. She withered away to a mere 86 lbs. She has lost all desire to be fit or healthy. She was a walking skeleton. Myla realized she needed to be back home.

She ended her college career at East Tennessee State University and moved home to Indiana. Unfortunately, while the signs were all there that Myla was suffering from an eating disorder; her family thought she was using drugs. Her mother had always been the type to make sure she was presentable. Her hair was always done, her clothes pressed and her nails done. Regardless of why Myla looked the way she did, the end result was her mother was embarrassed by her daughter's appearance. She couldn't understand how someone could look so bad willingly. It is hard to accept that something as simple as "not eating" could be the problem with your child. Obviously, the disorder goes much deeper than that.

While she was in the throes of this horrible affliction, Myla happened across a church camp that was in need of volunteer counselors. In hindsight, she laughs thinking that a person who was as wracked with her own personal problems could be seen as one to help others. Yet it is often the one who hurts the most who can help the most. Perhaps the group saw their partnership was not only Myla helping them, but them helping Myla. Either way, the time with the church camp worked wonders.

Obviously, one short summer helping a couple of kids did not turn Myla's life around completely. But it did help her start to get on track. Finding a purpose in helping others allowed her to help herself. She began to eat healthier again. She was exercising more, now that she had the energy. She knew she was far from out of the forest. Anyone who knows anything about anorexia can attest that it only takes a little to backslide into danger. She began to see the light at the end of the tunnel but sometimes wondered if it belonged to a train barreling down at her.

She began to do research. She was trying to find programs which could lend some assistance to those with anorexia. At the same time she was still battling her old habits. Her weight dipped into the double digits again. One day she happened across a program at Iowa State University that was tailored specifically for those with eating disorders. She thought given her history she would be an ideal candidate. You can imagine how dumbfounded she was when she was turned down. Perhaps she wasn't yet thin enough?

Fortunately, it did not take long for her to learn exactly why she had not been allowed into the program. A doctor who helped administer this organization had taken one look at Myla and told her a program could not help. She needed to go to the hospital immediately. She was too far past any program at any college and he feared for her life. When Myla informed her mother of what the doctor had told her, her mother cried and said nothing. To this day, she doesn't know exactly why her mother couldn't handle her daughter asking for help. All she knew was that she had to take on another set of difficult life changes without the support of her family.

The hospital she finally went to was in Des Moines. Her stay saved her life. She was ridiculously thin, just a whisper of a human. Yet the veil had been lifted from her eyes and she could see the problem for what it was. She was dealing with it the best way possible.

It was a long time before she was even trusted to monitor her own weight and health. But this is where running became her saving grace. If she didn't eat, she didn't have the energy to run. If she didn't run, she wasn't happy. Therefore, eating meant happiness for the first time in her life. The elation she felt from being stronger and fitter felt better than anything else. It was more than enough to keep her on the straight and narrow.

She worked on her running over the course of years. Her mileage increased and she took on longer and longer races. In 2003, she finally worked her mileage up to take on the Chicago Marathon. Her goal was to break four hours. She missed that by running a 4:19 but knew how much she had overcome to get to this point and how impressive that was. Yet she wanted more. She wanted to show how she could be both a person battling a disease and a strong woman at the same time. She would not play the victim. She would not let the disease beat her. Myla set her sights on the 2005 Marine Crops Marathon, which would happen right near her 40th birthday. She felt this would be a perfect way to culminate all her hard work and throw in some birthday cake as well. During her training she did smart thing one should do as they get over the age of 40. She got a mammogram.

While Myla does not like to call herself a cancer survivor, the fact remains that what doctors found on the mammogram were pre-cancerous cells. The small cluster of cells, if left inside of her, would have assuredly developed into cancer. So she had them removed. She wasn't done fighting yet. Having battled through so much she went back to what helped her most when she was having difficulty. Helping others.

Myla found herself moving to the greater Dallas, Texas area. While the sum total of what she had survived was rather unique, she knew many of the individual difficulties in her life were shared by others. She wanted to take the life lessons she had learned and do what she could in order to help others who were going through similar troubles. Giving back is what made Myla tick. So, like that plucky 7th grade girl who helped create her own track team, Myla started the North Oak Cliff Morning Running Group.

As weight loss is often a major motivator for many taking on running, Myla thought she would serve as a cautionary tale to others that too thin is not healthy. She would applaud the effort of those trying to get into better shape but she would also make sure the pendulum did not swing too far the other way.

To further her involvement with her local running area, Myla became the Activities Coordinator for the North Texas Trail Runners, a trail running group with over 500 members. Her involvement with so many groups was one done almost out of necessity for her own health and well-being. She surrounds herself with people who are having a tough time because often those people are excellent at giving help themselves. They might not seek out, receive, or even help themselves very well, but they are the ones who need it the most. Combining the sport of running, where people can lean on each other and draw from their collective strength, only seemed to make sense. Myla continues to need that strength to this day.

You see, during this time of growth and healing, Myla lost another close friend in another tragic way. Her friend was climbing Mt. Hood in Oregon when the unthinkable happened: he fell. His body was never recovered and the pain of never having closure to that event reminded her that her eating disorder would never go away. Once again, she yo-yoed in and out of dealing with bad habits as this crushing blow to her psyche was gnawing at her. But this time, her involvement with others helped keep her stable. She knew others were depending on her. She had to stay strong.

Looking back, she realized running helps her cope. It always has. She loves the camaraderie of running but she also likes to be by herself. As her running pursuits have gotten longer and she has found her way into ultramarathons, she finds herself running solo a great deal. Well, solo in the sense that no other humans are around her. Running alone is often what happens during an ultramarathon. Runners spread out for miles and miles and you are often that single solitary spec out in the wilderness. But this is where Myla talks to the people she has lost. She uses this time to come to grips with her own demons and face them with the spirit of a runner. She reflects on the good times in her life and shares them with the people who used to be a part of it.

Myla continues to push forward as a survivor against not only the miles in a race, but also the miles of her life. The blows she has been dealt would lay flat many others and often have taken her to her knees. But with her inner fire and what she has both taken and given from her sport, she pushes forward.

Besides, each finish line is just another starting line.

8

Annie Burke

Annie Towanda has employed running to assist her in reforming her body to be the crutch which she leaned on during an incredible personal struggle, and now she plans on using it to pay her bills. She is happy with where her journey has taken her and how she came out in the end. However, even if she had known her life would lead her to where she is happy, that knowledge would not have made living through it much easier.

Growing up in New Jersey, Annie was overweight. Actually, she was obese. At barely 5'2" she tipped the scales at 180 pounds. Her father, a retired lieutenant colonel in the Air Force, found dealing with life out of the service to be difficult. As with many who have thought alcohol is the answer, he crawled inside of a bottle. Annie's mother couldn't handle this and moved to Florida without her husband and without her children. This left Annie and her siblings to more or less fend for themselves. Most of her early life was spent in and out of foster care.

Strikingly poor, Annie did what she could to get by. This usually meant she would eat whatever food she could get hands on whenever she could. There was no saving food for tomorrow when it was placed in front of her. When you don't necessarily know when your next meal will be coming and whose home it will be at, you have a tendency to pack it away.

In addition to her weight problem, her chronic asthma led to difficulty with even trying to exercise. She never once took a gym class, always finding ways to get out of physically asserting herself. Combining an overweight kid with the inability or simple lack of a desire to exercise is a recipe for disaster. Yet, Annie wanted to get better.

In spite of what she saw from her father, she felt the military was the way to go for a better life. The Air Force seemed like a great opportunity for her to not only lose weight but also get her out of a less than enviable position in life. Unfortunately, she could not pass the medical exam. Her weight was a problem but she knew she could shed the unwanted pounds. But her asthma was simply too much. With no money and no real future in much of anything, she was left with few options. Where life appeared to be taking her did not look like someplace she wanted to be.

Fortunately for Annie, in spite of all the troubles, which made learning hard for so many underprivileged children, her grades were good enough to get her into college. From there she began to do what she could in order to make ends meet. While the military wouldn't accept her, she had law enforcement in her blood. She might not have been very fit, but she had a sense of right and wrong. She decided she would become a police officer.

At the tender age of nineteen she found an agency in Florida that would hire her. However, she only had a nine-month window to get into the physical condition they would accept. So she started running.

This being in the middle of the 1980s, there was no internet for Annie to turn to in order to find support. There were no online training plans for her to follow. She simply sloughed off to the library and began checking out books on the sport. She threw everything she had into running and learning how to take control of her weight and her health.

Before long she was running five miles a day. Her asthma was still a problem but she battled through it. Running helped lessen the load both figuratively and literally as the weight came off. For seven months she ran every day. Her end goal was not just a better healthful version of herself but an escape as well. The law enforcement agency job would be her ticket to a better life. When the only train out of town is one that requires you to run to it, you lace up your shoes.

She lost the weight and got the job.

Her first detail was working security at Trump Plaza. After some time defending the Tower which Bad Hair Built, she joined the police academy. The fat girl who never took a gym class soon became the number one female in her class. She had transformed herself from roly-poly into a fit woman who was ready to tackle the rigors of being a cop. Annie realized that in order to handle the toughness of the job, she had to be tougher. Three years on the force kept her in prime physical condition. Then the sheriff's office and some of the most tumultuous times of her life came calling.

For twenty-four years, Annie called the sheriff's office, specifically the Internal Affairs department, her home and life. Her co-workers became family. She worked her way up to the rank of captain and was the highest ranking woman in the agency. Unfortunately and mostly unbeknownst to her, she had ruffled feathers by simply doing the only thing she knew how to do: work hard.

An opportunity arose for her to take a three-month class in the FBI in the greater DC area. She didn't really need the job to help her advancement but it was definitely a feather in her cap. Annie had already made huge strides in her life, but there was nothing wrong with a few more. As the second oldest child she had already seen three of her siblings die from drug overdoses. Her father had abandoned the family in favor of the bottle. Her mother abandoned the family by moving away. Annie simply wanted to show she belonged. She wanted to show herself she was worth the effort and would not stop.

At the FBI academy class it was a cold winter. Going from class to class in between buildings was like getting hit with an artic wind. At one point shuttling herself between two classes was just too much for her asthma. She forgot that in cold weather it would flare up something awful. Having lived in Florida for more than two decades she rarely had to deal with any problems. But here, in the north, was a different situation entirely.

As the coughing grew stronger and her breathing more irregular, Annie knew she had to get inside. It might be a stretch to say it was a matter of life and death but not by much. In order to get into this government building on her way back to her dorm, Annie had to go through a checkpoint. This checkpoint did not allow person to carry guns through. Annie forgot she had her registered firearm in her purse. Carrying a gun like this in her purse was not at all uncommon for most female officers. She knew it was a mistake and figured to get a reprimand for failing to remember where her firearm was at all times. Instead of a slap on the wrist, however, she was expelled from the FBI program and sent packing.

In shock, she drove home to Florida. She figured there had to have been a mistake with her being expelled. Someone must have gotten some fact mixed up in the whole thing. But on the long drive home she had plenty of time to think. She started to put two and two together and figured out what exactly had transpired.

Annie was not only the highest ranking female in her agency but was also the highest ranking female in her position in the internal affairs office. The often looked-down upon branch of the police department that keeps the rest of the police officers from becoming corrupt, Annie had become accustomed to being given the cold shoulder by some of her fellow officers. But would their distaste for her position be so great as to cut her career off at the knees for such a small infraction?

Back in Florida, she expected to work everything out. Instead, she was put on administrative leave. No reason was given for why this was done but Annie knew she was being targeted. Everything she had worked so hard for was being taken away from her. She became so stressed she essentially stopped eating. She kept exercising but wasn't putting any fuel in the furnace. She started to shrink and wither. The once obese girl was sliding the other direction and rapidly finding herself in danger of dying from being too thin. The last time she weighed herself she barely registered 88 pounds. She knew she needed to find an outlet. The girl who turned to running to make her thinner now turned to it once again to bring her back from being too thin.

She knew she needed to be fit because she had to be strong. She had to be strong because she was fighting a battle for everything she had struggled to achieve. Life was not about to get any easier in the upcoming months. For her small infraction, Annie was demoted two ranks. This was the first time in the history of the department that anyone had ever been dropped two complete ranks. Yet she could not get an answer from anyone as to why these decisions were being made against her. Her hand was forced to take the matter through the appropriate legal channels. She never wanted to go against the job that had been part of her life for a quarter of a century, but it was evident that life was now against her. So she fought back.

For four years, Annie fought against this unjust and unexplained vendetta. During that time her running made her stronger. She grew to love the sport. Her weight returned. Her strength grew. She found herself running a marathon. Then another. While she fought against the system determined to bring her down, Annie ran 78 marathons. Obviously the system picked the wrong girl with whom to mess.

Finally, in January 2012, the case was settled out of court. Annie was reinstated to her previous position with full honors. She then promptly retired. While she is unable to talk about the exact specifics of the case, Annie does feel she was targeted because of her involvement as an Internal Affairs officer. She never once thought that the distaste for the office ran as deep as it obviously did. Or maybe some felt she gained too much. Perhaps it was a sexist thing. Maybe others didn't like how far she had pulled herself up by her own bootstraps. There is a possibility of a myriad of reasons why events unfurled as they did. Yet Annie does not hold a grudge. While the tumultuous period made her death defyingly thin it also brought her closer to the sport she loves.

After retiring, Annie began working for the State of Florida in Jacksonville. But she missed running. During her fight against her old job, the friends she had once made in the academy had been replaced by other friends-the ones she made out on the roads and trails. These were friends who not only didn't care what your position or rank was, they often didn't even know what your "real" job was. All they cared about was if you showed up Saturday morning at the agreed upon time to go run a hard 18 miler. These friends were the new family for Annie. Quite possibly the best family she ever had.

As long back as 2009, Annie had thought about opening a running store. As the pressure of the crucible that was the fight against the academy intensified, she realized more and more how much she wanted to control her own destiny. In running, we are given a set of genes from our parents. We can't control how many fast twitch or slow twitch muscle fibers we are given. But we can control what we do with those. Annie wanted to control what she could. So, she decided to leave the job she had and pursue her own dream.

In September of 2014, Annie opened her running store. She now has a life that enriched and fulfilled her like no other before. She could spend her days around the people who meant the most to her. No longer is she taking down criminals. No longer does she have to fight a system which wished to bring her down. Now she takes down shoe sizes. Her only fights are those metaphoric ones against the wall in a marathon and beyond.

Annie is 62 inches of dream-chasing machine who shows that while the end is not determined, the way we deal with how we get there definitely is.

9

Women's Running Today

Earlier we gave you a history of women's running and how we got to where we are today. More accurately, we told you how we got to the mid 90's. While that might seem like it was just the other day, the sport for females has evolved so much in the past two decades. It is a shame how little women know what has happened to their sport since then. To put it in perspective, if you are a 20 year old in 2014, you will have never known a race that could not be electronically chip-timed. Yes, the Champion Chip made its debut at the Berlin Marathon in 1994. So, obviously, while where women have been in the distant past is important, where they are today bears much delving into.

We undoubtedly celebrate and will point out some more feminine aspects of the changes that have been made by female runners in the last twenty years. Yet we bristle at many of the "milestones" we found reported on by newspapers, magazines and the like. Women can be just as competitive and seeking of victory as men. So to "pinkify" everything women runners do these days does a drastic disservice to all the pioneers who strive to keep women from being seen as just a frillier version of their male counterparts.

For example, according to Running USA's 2013 Marathon Report, women have gone from being just 11% of all marathon finishers in 1980 to 42% in 2012. In all races nationwide of all distance, it appears women actually outnumber male finishers. But this didn't just happen overnight. It took a few innovators, thousands of followers and many pairs of shoes.

Not long after Oprah crossed that finish line of the Marine Corps Marathon in 1994, social worker and Hawaii Ironman triathlete Molly Barker started working on a project. Her project was to create an organization that helped lay the groundwork for strong women by making strong girls. In 1996 she founded Girls on the Run with the goal of helping girls from 3rd through 8th grade gain self-confidence by training for a 5K. Starting with just thirteen students in Charlotte, North Carolina, the program soon spreads to 173 cities across North America with over 100,000 participants.

Projects like Barker's have 18 years later, put forth an entire generation of female runners. More importantly, they have fostered an inner strength among women to show them what can be done. Even if most of the girls don't run at an elite level, or even run much at all later in life, the seeds sown in programs that reach out to women at a youthful level can be seen growing in women today. Community leaders, entrepreneurs and those who push the boundaries would rarely be able to do so if they had not at least had the support at the youngest level.

When it comes to pushing boundaries, ultra-runner Pam Reed has shown she can hang with the boys, and then beat all of them. In 2002, Pam won the Badwater Ultramarathon, a 135-mile course that snakes through Death Valley in the middle of July when temperatures soar to 120 degrees. When she crossed the finish line, she did not simply beat all the females in the race, but all of the competitors.

Pam's victory set many things in motion in the ultra-running world, including tons of studies which seem to point to how women may actually be better suited to run very long distances than their bigger, stronger male counterparts. Whether this may be true in the end is not of consequence. The mere fact it is being discussed and entertained as a possibility shows the strides that have been made in the field of women's running.

While ultra-running can be seen to be populated a bit by a tough-as-nails, hardier women (not the case but definitely a public perception held by some), extreme events can be done by those who exude femininity. In 2004, Nicole Deboom took on the grueling 140.6 mile Ironman Wisconsin. When she bested all of her competitors wearing a running skirt, eyebrows were raised. Later that year she founded her own company designing and selling these skirts.

You will often hear that women were told many decades ago, that if they ran too much there was a likelihood that their uterus would fall out. We like to laugh and point at those bygone times and think of ourselves as so much more enlightened. The fact of the matter is that no one of any reasonable sense or scientific mind actually thought those things. (Similar attributions have been given to how if any person ever ran under 4 minutes for a mile, they would die. No one believed that but it makes good copy, as they say.)

However, how hard women could push themselves, especially if they were thinking about or had recently had a child was up for debate. Given women hadn't been allowed to do so, at least publically, meant there was something to be discovered. When Paula Radcliffe, she of the 2:15 marathon World Record decided to run the New York City Marathon in 2007, just 10 months after giving birth to her first child, here was a situation ripe with possibilities.

Radcliffe had famously famed out of the 2004 Athens Olympic Marathon, crashing and burning on the curb just 3 miles from the finish. The British press had destroyed her in the papers about giving up and not being strong enough. The tones of the articles were thinly veiled but obviously were pointing to the fact that a man would not have done something of this sort. Here was the best marathoner ever, sobbing on the side of a road when if she had just walked the final 3 miles she would still have had a time most runners couldn't dream of running.

In other words, the greatest female marathoner ever was still being treated like a little girl. But Paula not only went on to win the Marathon, she did it one second faster than her 2004 victory with the second fastest winning time by a woman in the race's history. Then the next year she came back and won it again. I guess mothers can run.

In the half a decade or so since that victory by Radcliffe, women's running has again jumped leaps and bounds in different ways. Elite female times have stagnated a touch with hardly anyone coming within sniffing distance of Radcliffe's mark of 2:15:25 set in 2003. However, the time she set has come under criticism. In 2011, right years after she set the mark, the International Association of Athletics Federations, which is the international governing body for the sport of athletics, declared Radcliffe's time to be not a world record but a world best. The reasoning? Radcliffe ran the London race with male pacemakers, which the IAAF says makes for an unfair edge compared to all-women races. How that made sense was anyone's guess but it was another fight that women had to take on. Fortunately, this caused quite a kerfuffle and not only amongst female competitors.

Finally the IAAF had to relent and grandfather (mother?) in Radcliffe's record and say that only future events which vied to be world records would have to be done in women-only events. This has still left a great distaste in the mouths of many, as it appears to be another slight toward female athletes. Almost a handholding if you will of how the poor girls can't compete their hardest if the big burly men don't lead the way. This, of course, ignores the proven fact that it is easier for any gender to run harder when they have people pushing them.

But if anything, the IAAF's decision as ludicrous as it was, and the people who responded to it, shows that women have made huge strides in the running world. While they may be slighted by some governing body or some apparel company or whomever, the response does not take months or years to remedy the situation. It is immediate and forceful. The silver lining is becoming a silver cloud.

Women are now currently the vanguard for some major changes in our sport. Traditionally, shoe companies were the biggest sponsors for the elites trying to make a living at running. You signed with a shoe company and whatever apparel came with that shoe company came with it. However at the beginning of 2014 Kara Goucher, one of the two major recognizable faces of American running, left Nike after 12.5 years.

The reasons were many but her own. The end result was that Goucher ended up with Giselle, a running apparel company based out of Seattle, as her major sponsor. Not a shoe company as has been what runners have strived for since they were allowed to seek sponsorships, but a smaller female-owned apparel company. No male runner of note had made such a bold move. Perhaps, men don't need to think less traditionally in these arenas as women do. Perhaps it is simply a harbinger of where the world of sports and the economy is heading. Regardless, the trailblazing for the future has started today.

And the hacking of the underbrush is being done by women.

10

Holly Koester

If you want to feel weird for feeling sorry for someone with a disability, meet Holly Koester. One shouldn't normally have remorse about extending a feeling of sorrow for those who seemingly have it harder than the rest of us. If anything, the emotion shows compassion and good will. It is a natural reaction to see someone who has suffered a loss of some normal function, be it walking or sight or anything we all take for granted, and say something along the lines of "Well, that sucks for them." Empathy is wonderful. However, spending just five minutes with Holly in her wheelchair will make you not only never feel sorry for her again, but will instantly remind you how lucky you are and how little you are taking advantage of your good fortune.

Holly was born in Buffalo, New York and is naturally a Buffalo Bills fan. One would think that suffering along with that team would give the fates pause in dealing out more pain and suffering. How much can one person handle, really? But if there ever was a person seemingly suited to deal with setback, even one that will change every single aspect of their life, it is Ms. Koester.

Holly joined the Reserve Officers' Training Corps (ROTC) in college with her twin sister mainly to get a scholarship. She was aware of the dangers of the world and how she might be called upon to serve her country by doing so. Like most people who joined the service, she thought nothing of it. The only people who get hurt are others. She was happy to do what she could to help her country and have it help put her through school.

A natural athlete growing up, Holly played softball and soccer and balanced it with some track in high school. In college, she took up volleyball. When she was in the ROTC and later the Army she added softball back into the mix. All the sports involved running to some extent and she was fine with huffing it up and down the field. That is what legs are meant to do after all – be in motion.

For ten years Holly served her country without incident or thought to how fortunate she was to be able to go for a run. While at Redstone Arsenal in Alabama, Holly was in an auto accident on post. Now a captain, Holly, who had already marched a few marathons of her own through drills, knew she was in trouble. Her vehicle had flipped over on her and pinned her to the ground. By the time she got to the hospital it did not take doctors long to see she had completely severed her spinal cord at the T-7 level? The weekend after Desert Storm had been declared in the Gulf, Holly was now a paraplegic. She would never run, let alone walk again.

For seven days Holly was in the hospital while doctors tried to stabilize her spine. They were hoping that no further damage would occur, completely paralyzing her. Placed in a Stryker frame, her body was immobilized in a circular tube of pipes and bolts. She was rotated slowly, primarily to make sure bedsores did not complicate matters. Often being hung facing the floor, strapped to her bed, Holly's perspective, like her life, was turned upside down. Her mother, who rarely left her side, would simply slide in under her, like a mechanic looking at a carburetor, and have a chat with her for a bit. When Holly recounts what has to be a very difficult memory of this time you never hear a woe is me tone in her voice. There is no sadness as to what she lost or searching for blame. Instead, you are laughing along with her as she recounts the oddity of the situation and how weird it was for everyone involved. Her attitude is simply amazing.

When she finally left the hospital, Holly had to choose where she would take on her rehabilitation. Since her rehab would basically be an ongoing event for the rest of her life, she was in turn also choosing her home base for eternity. The hospital that offered the most, and was as close to her family as possible, was in the greater Cleveland area. So, to the Buckeye State Holly went. Fortunately, her support system was very strong and uprooted itself to where they could provide her with the utmost of care and love. There is never a second in which you doubt how grateful Holly is that she has a family which has supported her as well as hers has.

After barely being in her new digs for three months, Holly entered herself in the National Wheelchair Games. She was progressing about as well as anyone could have hoped. Entering the games and taking on the challenge they presented was what made sense to her. She knew no other way but to move forward. Rather than go the easy route, Holly decided the slalom, a challenging obstacle course, would be the first event she would try. It was only later in the games when she saw a woman going around the track repeatedly that she thought of entering a standard distance "footrace." Her first event saw Holly not in any sort of racing wheelchair, with smooth tires and aerodynamic placement, but rather her normal, ramrod-straight, manual chair with hard plastic tires.

The races and the miles piled up. Holly found she enjoyed pushing herself in this manner and it helped her keep her positive attitude. She traded in her regular wheelchair and was able to upgrade to the sleeker low-profile wheelchairs we are used to seeing today. This chair wasn't all carbon fiber and helium wheels but she was at least no longer pushing a Buick around. With the effort required to push this wheelchair less than before, she thought perhaps she could go much further. The last race she had completed as an able-bodied runner was the Indy Mini Marathon. She felt this would be the perfect place to make her debut at the 13.1 distance. Crossing the finish line was an emotional one for her. Even the positive mental capacity she had such a firm grasp on could crack in emotional times. Crossing a line, which she had previously crossed on two legs, was something that really stuck with Holly for a while.

For that reason, and a few more, Holly waffled at the idea of taking on a full 26.2-mile race. There was no doubt she was determined to do things on her own as much as possible though in the meantime. She had the handles from the back of her chair removed so people would not be tempted to assist her in getting around. Besides the autonomy this gave her and how much it forced her to really do things under her own power she also mentioned it was a major relief. As well meaning as the action of helping someone in a wheelchair is, imagine how terrifying it must be to suddenly have the object you are sitting in, suddenly be no longer under your control. So Holly decided to nip that in the bud.

She continued to race, often staying as close to home as possible. At an event one weekend, she met Paralympian Jean Driscoll. She had some long talks with her about dealing with the changes in one's life which come from once being ambulatory and now having little to no use of your legs. Jean, born with spina bifada, but who did not use a wheelchair until high school, really touched a chord with Holly. Here was someone in her own situation doing what she hesitated to pull the trigger on. So, she decided to take that next step. The Columbus Marathon would be her first ever in a wheelchair. Now, the question was no longer if she would someday take on the marathon but rather an exact date and time. She was committed.

After completing the Columbus Marathon, Holly now began a new plan. She wanted to take on every single one of the military marathons. She also wanted to use her new found goals as a reason to see some interesting cities across the United States. At the Houston Marathon, she ran into the booth for the 50 States Marathon club. This club is one which celebrates those who try to complete as many marathons in as many states as possible. While going to every state had not previously been on her radar she thought it sounded like an excellent idea. She signed up for the club on the spot and began wheeling.

From Florida to Maine to Hawaii to Alaska where she finally completed the 50 States circuit, Holly rolled on. Now,

133 marathons later, Holly is the first and only wheelchair athlete to have completed a marathon in all 50 states. She not only was able to get those 50 states (and so many other marathons in between) but she also did them all in a push-rim wheelchair. Considered to be far more difficult than the hand-crank style, Holly felt it best approximated "running" for her. She knew she would never use her legs again but by adding this challenge within a challenge, she felt she was pushing her boundaries as far as possible.

Only recently has Holly allowed herself to use a hand crank wheelchair on occasion. All the miles of racing and training were finally starting to take a toll on her shoulders. She realized that with her legs already gone, the last thing she needed was to lose her own means of mobility by destroying her shoulders as well. So much to her chagrin, and almost against her own code, the hand crank chair occasionally made an appearance at races. She hopes to keep those shoulders as fresh as possible for as long as she can. She definitely has no plans to stop racing. She may be more cautious but her drive and fevered determination are just as strong as ever.

Outside of the racing world, Holly has obviously had to make change to her daily life. The simplest of tasks when she was able to walk have now become difficult to impossible. Runners often joke about how the things they talk about with regards to their own personal hygiene would shock others. Which is why it should be of no surprise conversations with Holly will lead to discussions about the basic needs in life which many of us never give a second thought. As a paralyzed person, Holly doesn't go to the bathroom the same way that you and I do. She can sometimes predict when she will need to use the bathroom but often it is hit and miss. She mentions how when she was still taking classes, she often would have to throw pants away and put on some clean ones. She wasn't about to carry soiled pants from class to class all day.

Even when the dirty details are handled there still remains the matter of being able to reach things. Imagine always being in a seated position trying to reach up for things in a world not designed for you. Those with some vertical challenges are the best at understanding how this is but the worst-case scenario for them is to drag a footstool from one place to another in their home. Holly says her roommates laugh because now all the dishes are down low. Even more so, because of her limited reach, Holly actually had to redesign her whole kitchen. She completely lowered one counter so she could chop vegetables and mix food or even just use it as a counter. She also realized how non-accessible her house was in general. Getting into many rooms, including the bathroom was impossible. The wheelchair simply wouldn't fit. So bring out the contractor. You're going to need a bigger door.

When she is shopping, she becomes painfully aware of all the essentials that are kept up high. Butter, milk, bread, cleaning supplies, medicines and cereals are just a few things placed usually out of the reach of children for safety's sake. Unfortunately, they are also out of the reach of someone in a wheelchair. Holly has so many instances where something she wants is just a fingernail's length out of reach. Just a fraction of an inch between her and what she wants but it might as well be a mile.

Holly thinks runners can understand the dilemma of fractions of an inch better than anyone. Because we often deal in such minute details, seconds on the clock, or tenths of a second if we are sprinters, are very comparable to the items just out of her reach. Many times, Holly will think she has something in her hand and at the last moment, the wrong movement will push it further away. Often she will use other objects to knock something down into her hand. She uses tools she has learned which will make her life easier. If you are beginning to see similarities between the fractions of inches from Holly's groceries to her fingertips and your own running goals, this is not an accident.

Street curbs were once invisible. Now they are the biggest headaches. A step here or there she never noticed in her house now have to be dealt with as if it were a mountain. Outside her home, the world became an obstacle course. Granted, the United States in particular has become much more user-friendly for those with disabilities such as Holly's, but it is still a tough life even for those with the best of attitudes. Yet somehow Holly smiles and pushes forward.

Her countenance and smile can light up any room. You hear no self-pity in her voice whatsoever. She speaks with a matter-of-factness that puts you at ease with her situation. When asked how she can stay so upbeat when so much as taken away from her, she thinks of her time spent at Walter Reed Medical Hospital. She speaks of soldiers who have lost all mobility or their sight or their hearing. "It's not hard to see others who have it must worse than me. That always helps me keep it in perspective."

If only we all had that attitude.

11

Laura Frey

Runners often see those at the front of the pack as being bereft of worry. The speedsters have so much fastness in their legs that even a bad day for them is one mere mortals would "give anything to run". Failure for a 4-minute per mile runner is to run a 4:20. Their speed and strength is so otherworldly that they are not seen as actual flesh and blood. They are just "those people". Yet their worries and fears are just the same as those who run much slower. In fact, if they don't hit their goals, more people tend to be critical of their performance. They don't have the luxury of "just finishing". However, some relish this added pressure. They do not mind being looked at under a microscope. Turning on the light just makes them shine even more. Laura Frey, who ran her first marathon in a 3:02, was not one of those who loved the pressure being on her.

Growing up in Portsmouth, New Hampshire, there was never really a question of whether Laura was fast. Unlike many runners today, Laura did not see running as punishment. For as long as she can remember, she liked to run. Coupled with her love for the sport was how good she was at it. However, even in elementary school if you are the fastest around you are going to get attention. Laura did not like it.

She loved running hard and fast on the track. Sweating and feeling the pain deep in her thighs was her way of experiencing life. She liked to be competitive and push herself and others. She liked to win. If she could have found a way to race against competitors, give her all and then disappear, that would have been ideal. But no such way existed. So she hung up her track shoes.

When high school approached, she thought perhaps her fear of being in the limelight had faded. She knew her love for running had not. So she thought she would give the organized portion of the sport she loved so much another go. Joining the cross-country team, she loved the feeling of the wind on her face. The grass under her feet was her own little high. The rush of endorphins was more than enough to please her. Unfortunately, the rigorous structure of practice and training was not her bag. In spite of her talent, the love for this portion of the sport did not exist. So, once again she called it quits.

When she went to college in Miami she never once thought about joining the athletics squads in Coral Gables. Athletics is a religion in Miami. She knew if she did not like the spotlight in New Hampshire, she assuredly couldn't stand it at the "U". So instead she simply lived her life as a normal student, did well in her classes and graduated. She kept in shape by exercising on her own terms. Yet in spite of staying in shape, she ached to run again. Once again she hopped back on the familiar horse.

She started by hitting the treadmills in local gyms. She couldn't stand the running in soup atmospheric conditions. Also, unlike now where the running scene has exploded in Miami, when she lived there it was still in its beginning stages. As such, she had few partners to choose from and even less desirable places to run. Nevertheless, in spite of the time off she could tell she still had some speed in her legs.

At age 30, she moved to North Carolina with her new husband. While the heat and humidity are still present in the Tarheel State there are also forests to run through. Trails beckoned there. She never really had any plan to race or get competitive again. She simply wanted to run, solo, on her own terms, with no teammates. Just the way she liked it.

Every day she laced up her shoes and found herself lost in the Carolina wilderness. There was no pressure and no coaches with clipboards and whistles. No bibs to pick up and no competitors to race. But even as pleasing as this was, she felt maybe she did want more. Perhaps shirking structure and rigid practice as a youth was finally out of her system. Here is where Laura finally made the decision to race.

Her workouts grew with intensity. The composition of her training became more focused. She started to circle dates on the calendar for important upcoming races. Her attention was now turned toward facing her fears of the spotlight. She would fine-tune her body to be the missile it was meant to be. Of course, pregnancy can throw all of that off a bit.

Having twins was not going to stop Laura now that her fire was stoked. Under her doctor's care she continued to run for as long as she could. She knew that her health and well-being meant her children would be healthy as well. So she continued to run while her hopeful future runners grew inside of her. She finally stopped running only when her stride became affected by her belly. After neglecting her love of running for so long, she knew it was prudent to not injure herself with an unnatural gait. Yet she knew as soon as she could after giving birth she would want to run again. So Laura took this down time to research jogging strollers. These babies were going to grow up seeing the world 7 minutes per mile at a time.

Soon after they were born, Isabella and Sophia were in that stroller. Her daughters now jokingly tell their mother that their first memories are of wiping off sweat that dripped from her chin onto them. Before long she was back into prime shape. She hadn't really set her schedule to pinpoint an exact race and get down to training for it before she found herself pregnant again. This time, her son Julian would be the one putting her racing plans on pause for a bit. But just like his sisters, he too soon saw the world as a blur in front of his mom.

Her drive and determination lead to her joining the North Carolina Roadrunners Club. Her litany of solo runs didn't change very much but now she had a dash of running friends thrown in as well. These runners supported her desire to race and compete. They helped her get over her anxiety about competition. They helped create a racing monster.

Nearly every weekend she found herself at the starting line of yet another 5k. Calling her a weekend warrior would denote her races were fun affairs and not the prize of a hard week of training. But now that Laura had found her stride again, nothing could be further from the truth. She relished her hard workouts and loved brining everything she had to race day. Age group wins became commonplace. Winning was something she was used to doing but now it felt good to be recognized for her efforts.

For quite some time she was content with the short distance stuff. She wasn't an ace at the 5k but ran fast enough to do fairly well. Mostly, racing satisfied a need and a desire. Laura knew she wasn't going to set the world afire with her short distance times but they were good enough for her. She also was setting a great example for her children on how to balance what needs to be done with what you would like to do. The importance of physical fitness was paramount to their upbringing.

She continued to race nearly every weekend but now the distances grew. Soon she set her sights on the marathon. By herself, with no coach, she targeted the Eugene Marathon in 2012 for her debut. On what she personally describes as "shit training" she ran a 3:02:41. She was hooked as you can imagine anyone would upon finishing in the top 10 of their gender in their first marathon. So she hired a trainer and began training even harder. Her work netted her two consecutive sub-3 hour finishes at Boston. She thinks she has a much faster time in her legs.

Her goals, in life, are to be motivated and to succeed. She wants to be a good mother. She hopes to show people what they can do in spite of their fears. Laura doesn't want others to let life be their excuse for not pursuing what they want. In order to do everything she has to do as a mother of three she gets up every day 4:55 am to go for her runs. She knows if she didn't love the sport this much how easily she could let it slip by the wayside. But she sure does love to run.

She loves the first mile. She loves the last mile. She loves going over her splits. Preparing for her next workout provides her with a balance so she can be the best version of herself in all facets of life.

She started a running blog because she wanted others to see about the changes she has made in her own life. Many now admire her dedication to the sport without knowing how often she gave it up. Her never give up attitude had to be cultivated over many years after, well, giving up frequently.

A few important people now found a love for the sport because of Laura: her children. Her twin daughters now enjoy some success of their own. Most recently Isabella made the State Finals of the Hershey Track and Field Games in North Carolina. Sophia and Julian are no slouches either. They love the competition and are anxious to run hard. They also don't exactly understand how every race can't be your best. When Laura recently took fourth place overall at the USATF master's 5,000-meter race (her first ever on a track) her kids were a little confused why she wasn't the winner.

So, running seems to have come full circle for Laura. A childhood wracked by the fear of succeeding now has her as a mother of three who want nothing more than to go full tilt. Laura has turned her own fears and anxiety into positives in hopes of inspiring others. Looking only at the end product, like her recent 4th place masters finish at the very hard Boilermaker 15k, one can think she is just all grit and talent.

Well, obviously the talent is there but the grit had to be earned.

And now Laura likes the pressure of earning it.

12

Michelle Niemeyer, Laura Hileman and Shannon Mitchel

Inspiration is defined as that which gives one a desire to do something or pushes them in the direction of creating or doing something. When writing a book about those who inspire the easy way out is to look for the stories which are traditionally put into the inspirational category. Without a doubt some of the more traditional inspirational women fill this book. The reasons why these people inspire are obvious. Those who have overcome odds after facing a devastatingly setback really tug on our heartstrings. As such, because these are the stories most likely to move us, we think that to be inspiring, someone has to have overcome a great obstacle. In other words, the truly inspirational must have been inflicted with a terrible disease, crushed by a horrible accident or been dealt a really rough hand in the card game of life. Unfortunately, this overlooks about 95% of human experience.

Many of us overcome obstacles that will never make an after-school special or be the subject of a moving article in a magazine. But because those obstacles are not of epic proportion does not mean they are inconsequential. The phrase "Well, in the grand scheme of things, my problems aren't all that bad" is often used to make light of a situation which seem dire at the time. This is a true statement. In the grand scheme of things, *no* problems are *that bad*. In fact, all problems are absolutely without mentioning if you want to go really grand in your scale-looking.

This is why, even though by nature, the stories of beating back the difficulties in life are the kind which move us, we have to remember and be inspired by those whose tales are much more indicative of the human struggle against daily life.

These are the tells of people who would have thoroughly enjoyed eating fatty food every single day but resisted. People with hardships that might not be Oprah-special worthy, are problems they still needed to handle. These are the women who were tempted by drugs, alcohol, crime or any other life-wrecking choice, but shoved that decision to the ground. Maybe they made a wrong decision here or there but they came out on the right side.

We live in an era of excuses. Many will point to a disorder, a lack of support from their family, or something else as to why they have not achieved what they hoped to achieve. Yet, we all know friends and family who refuse to allow excuses to determine their fate. While those who have bested their own bad decisions or fought back against cruel fate absolutely hold a place in our hearts, those who go through life doing things the right way also deserve recognition.

To the parents who have raised good children, not letting busy schedules stop them from finding time for exercise, play and the various activities for their kids, please take a bow. To the teens who refuse to allow the obesity "epidemic" claim them by taking time to eat right and exercise, the world is your oyster. If you have made the correct choices regarding drugs and alcohol, we are happy the future is in your hands. For everyone in between, who tackles adversity, fails, gets back up and soldiers on, this is, as Elton John sang, your song.

It may be boring to look at the person with the nice waistline, the good spouse and the nice smile and see them as inspirational. We may automatically assume a great deal has come easy to these people. However, chances are, the story of how they got to where they are now is just as inspiring as the ones we usually see leading the news. The women we highlight in this chapter have had their own hardships, let there be no mistake. We simply feel they too much be acknowledged.

**

Michelle Niemeyer decided she would take some time off from running. Eighteen years off, actually.

Being a high school runner paid off. She had run well enough in high school to get a scholarship to St. Xavier University. While in school, Michelle spent two years getting even faster posting some very solid times. Unfortunately, her parents moved out of state while she was still in college. As such, her state financial aid went with her parents in the U-Haul. Even with the scholarship she had from her cross-country running, she did not have enough to make ends meet. Her decision of staying in school was more or less made for her. With not enough money or financial aid to continue, Michelle had to drop out of college. No longer in school and now in the workforce, her running disappeared as well.

Fast forward to 2012. A high school friend messaged Michelle out of the blue about doing a mud run. The message was akin to something like "Hey, I remember you used to run. Come join us!" Michelle had not run since she had to make the decision about her future back at St. Xavier. At first she was embarrassed at the idea of joining her friends. She was no longer close to the running shape she had been when she clocked an 18:58 on a hilly cross-country 5k course in college. Now she was a mother of four girls and not exactly fit enough to take on run down the block, let alone any obstacle racing course. As she was only six months removed from her last child, there was really no reason for her take on this challenge. Of course, that means her friends immediately were able to talk her into doing so. In her own words:

"I remember that I had zip zero bladder control, horrible cramps, and no cardiovascular conditioning. Yet somehow when I crossed that finish I felt like a million bucks and couldn't wait to lace up again."

It didn't take Michelle long to convert her husband to be a runner as well. Even though their training schedules differ (someone has to watch the kids), she has someone who supports her training and races. She hasn't yet returned to the exact speed she had nearly two decades ago but she is getting closer. Even so, when she has a bad day, she knows her family will be there for her.

Recently she took on a half marathon, which was nearly two minutes per mile slower than her personal best. Feeling ornery and upset at her performance mid-race, her spirits were buoyed by her husband and children family waiting for her near the finish. Obviously she had not been having the best day but two of her daughters jumped in to run the last few miles with her.

She has had better days since then and continues to push for some more speed when she can. However, for Michele, showing her children to stick to your efforts, even when things do not look (or feel) that great, is a much better lesson than showing them how well you can do when everything is going wonderful. She feels that too often in life you will be called upon to act when few things are going your way. It is then which your character is truly revealed.

**

The love of running is often enough to attract many to the sport. Feeling the wind rush through your hair, blood pushing to the skin in your face as you push the envelope and the sweat dripping from temples is more than enough for most to catch the bug for running. Cute guys on the cross-country team doesn't hurt either.

Laura Hileman readily admits the opposite sex was a factor in her even taking on the sport in the first place in high school. But these boys weren't necessarily enough for her to fall in love with the sport. In fact, when she went onto college, running gave way to swimming. Post college, after getting married and having some children, she found herself busy and anxious. After seeing the prescription the doctor gave her to deal with this stress and anxiety, she felt there had to be a better way than medicating with these pills. So she self-medicated with a dose of asphalt and sweat.

She kept her running a secret, however. Her friends were completing in half-marathon and the like and she was amazed at the idea of anyone running 13.1 miles straight. She quietly enrolled in a Couch to 5k program to have guidance. She followed the training to the letter and found her anxiety and stress were relived. Laura's decision to see what was possible by adding exercise to her bloodstream far outperformed what taking some pills could have ever done. She found strength and resolve. In addition, she wanted to share this love with others.

Letting her friends know she was also a runner opened up a new world to her. They were excited for her to join the tribe and soon had her taking on different adventures of all distances. Her mileage increased and fifteen months after she started her journey, she took on her first half-marathon. Since then she had put seven more half marathons under her belt as well as an assortment of other races. She admits seeing the medals on the wall are often just the motivation she needs to get out the door. She doesn't necessarily race to get medals, but the physical manifestation of her hard work is never a bad thing.

Laura's running regiment has also expanded to her husband. Doing so has expanded their circle of friends. She calls her best friend her accountability partner and craves the time on the trails with her. As a mother of three, she finds these times she spends alone actually bring her closer to her family in the end. She comes back refreshed and ready to take on her role as a mother. With her husband running as well, they have become close friends with other running families. Laura and her group will plan trips, sometimes with her children and sometimes alone to race events across the country.

Now she stands on the cusp of taking on her first marathon. She feels her decision to take on running as an alternative way to help cure what ailed her has not only benefitted her in the long run but her children as well. Seeing that with hard work and good attitude your goals can be achieved has been paramount to helping her raise her children right. And there are some cuties running you want to chase, go right for it.

**

Some people decided to go back to school as an adult. Some even take some advances classes. Not many decide to completely change careers, change sport loves and reinvent themselves in their late 30s. Shannon Mitchel is not everyone.

After years spent chasing the acting and radio broadcast bug, Shannon was not happy with where she was. She enjoyed what she did and had starred in a few productions but she simply felt she was too typecast. She was always the cute girl next door but not tall enough to ever be the leading lady. After spending some time getting her physical therapist degree, Shannon also changed the way she exercised.

Having been a national champion baton twirler growing up, she had seen the country going on numerous tournament competitions. But she only saw the insides of gyms and auditoriums. She wanted to actually see the world now. Plus, because she was nowhere near as naturally talented running, she wouldn't have the same pressure. Furthermore, unlike twirling, there was no subjectiveness to her overall place. If she ran a half-marathon in 1:50, the Russian judge couldn't take that away on a technicality. Running was not done for sponsors or for her family. She did it for her.

Of course, going to medical school at age 38 is not the way to see much of anything but operating rooms, extremely thick text books, and almost never the backs of your eyelids. However, deciding you want to see the world 26.2 miles (or more) at a time sure is. Unfortunately, even with the drive and gumption of an unstoppable force, often life will still make things hard for you.

During medical school, Shannon got hit with a number of whammies. First her mother had a stroke. Then she got divorced. Finally her car up and died on her. Her federal loans were based on her being married and she simply couldn't take out any more money to deal with all of these at once. The expenses began to mount. Then, two months later when her mother died she had to take on additional private loans to handle the cost of burial. At this time she was knee deep in a very challenging general surgery residency. Unlike other residencies, this one does not allow a doctor to moonlight on the side to pay any additional bills. If you are short on money, you must simply take out more loans or have wealthy relatives. Shannon could not and did not have either. As such, she had no choice. She had to resign her residency.

She took a job as an as occupational medicine physician. Working her way up to surgeon she also began increasing her miles as a runner. Taking on marathons and ultramarathons is now relatively easy for someone who often went days without actually getting any real sleep. Shannon feels medical school was like a training camp for runners who want to learn how to keep moving when they are absolutely exhausted.

With a marathon personal best hovering just over four hours, Shannon knows she is not ever going to win a speed contest. But she has worked hard for every time she gets. Once, in a particular rocky and difficult 50-mile race, she fell and bashed her head. She is not sure how long she was unconscious and with no other runners around her in the ills at the time, it is difficult to tell. Fortunately, she got back to a place where she could quit the race and called it a day. Having worked the medical aid tent of many 100 milers, Shannon knew when it was time to stop.

By stop, we of course just meant for that race. It is quite clear that Shannon, like all of these every day women, knows very little about throwing in the towel over the long term. Their ability to do what they can with what they have at this very moment truly is the definition of inspiration. These women, like so many others out there, simply soldier on. They are not looking for awards for doing what they feel is what one simply must do. They just want a clearly marked course, some diet coke with ice and maybe a few hugs when they are done.

13

Luisa Miller

Luisa Miller thought about becoming a nun. Instead, she became a Marine.

Born and raised in Nicaragua until she was 6, Luisa knew from an early age that the path for females was linear. Grow up, have babies, go to the kitchen. That's the way life is in Central America if you happen to be female. Physical fitness is not only not a virtue, but time spent away from keeping the home in its pursuit is highly frowned upon. In our culture of equal rights and (at least the belief) of access to all for everyone, this seems appalling. For Luisa, it was simply life as she knew it. Women were largely meant to know their place (which was one of zero power and influence) and stay there.

Fortunately, for Luisa there was at least some hope. When she was young her family immigrated to Miami. She was now in the United States, where one could at least hope to break out of a centuries old patriarchal society reluctant to change. On the other hand, the insular nature of her neighborhood made it seem like there was no real difference between where she had come from and where she now resided. For all intents and purposes, she might have well been still living in Nicaragua. Women don't advance; they stay stagnant. Luisa still felt the pressure to conform to the standards of her native land. Those pressures, however, coupled with time, act like pressure does to those made of tough stuff: they make them stronger.

Luisa's path in Nicaragua had been one to be a nun. She felt it best fit her temperament. In addition, it offered the greatest opportunity to give her the highest standard of living as a woman. If her gender was considered second-class citizens, at least the top of that list were those in the black habits. She saw veiled power and security behind those cloaks. She knew the resolve and power one must have to take up a life of celibacy and devote their life to helping others. This seemed the admirable and intelligent way to try to live your life in a country that doesn't really respect you. Now, in America, she still wanted to help others, she saw other ways to do so.

In her last year of high school, a Marine recruiter came to Luisa's school. Virtually every person who came within earshot of this recruiter was asked whether they wanted to enlist to be one of the few and the proud. Luisa was blatantly ignored. Even the chubby out-of-shape boys who had trouble defending their waistlines were being asked to defend our borders. Flat out offended, Luisa didn't wait for the recruiter to approach her. Instead, she walked right up and asked why he hadn't even bothered with his pitch. Taken aback he made a special appointment just to see Luisa. She showed up but he did not. She had been stood up.

Undeterred she kept at it, finally cornering the recruiter. She asked him why he had not only ignored her in the first place but why he had also stood her up. In a matter of fact way, the recruiter told her it was nothing personal but in the eyes of the Marines at that time in that place, women were not seen as good recruits. Latin American women were seen as even less reliable. The thing about being told that something is not personal is that it rarely softens the blow of what follows next out of that person's mouth. Moreover, it is usually something deeply personal. This is where Luisa decided, if nothing else, she would show this recruiter this one Latin American woman was made of the right stuff.

Fast-forward and Luisa found herself deep into Marine Corps training. The nun had a new habit and it was running. Five days a week, for four years straight, her boots were on the ground moving forward. Feeling she already had two strikes against her by being both a Nicaraguan and a woman, she worked harder than most. Always running and giving everything her body could give was the path to earning and keeping the respect of her fellow Marines. The absolute last thing she desired was to be perceived as a weak link. She wanted her fellow Marines to think of her not as a girl or as a Central American but as one upon which they could rely. Having put in so much time and pride into even getting into the Marine Corps, the worst thing she could imagine was being unworthy of the eagle, globe, and anchor. These symbols, presented to all who graduated from three months of boot camp, were emblematic of everything she knew she could be.

So she trained. She ran. She suffered. The fear of needing to "fall out" of a long training run pushed her forward. They would have to drag her unconscious body off the course before she would endure the shame of stepping out of the military vehicle that picked her up because she couldn't hack it. Not moving forward became unthinkable. She refused to not keep up with her fellow Marines. IF they had to run through the heat and the muck and everything else, she was going to show all of them she could do the very same thing. She ran to survive, to prove herself to others, and to avoid embarrassment. Luisa also ran to cope.

Stationed at Camp Pendleton when the planes hit the Twin Towers in New York City, the Pentagon and a field in Pennsylvania, Luisa was in a formation run when she heard the sobering news. To this day, she claims to have never seen footage of that day or those planes crashing into American buildings and soil. The intensity is too much for her to bear. Coming to America meant getting away from crime and strife and violence. Even joining the Marines, where she knew she could be part of a bigger battle, was done as a means to an end. She was not shying away from her duties as a Marine, but she never thought about how the world could turn on a single day. So instead she buried herself in the running she loathed.

Running might have been something she did constantly, but it had never been something she enjoyed. It was simply what you did to belong to what you now were. But after that fateful day, running became cathartic. Putting one foot in front of the other was a release. It was when she was allowed to make decisions about her life, at least with regards to run she wanted to do. She couldn't control her surroundings. She couldn't control whether she was deployed. But she was the master of her own run.

However, sometimes dedication can only take you so far. In 2002, when her enlistment with the Marine Corps ended, she rebelled against running. While it had helped her through the tough times, it now reminded her of the things she did not want to think about. Running was not associated with forcing herself to forget. She did not want to remember that she was supposed to forget. So for nearly two years she barely ran at all. She got married and became pregnant. Running became a distant memory.

Ten months after giving birth to her daughter a co-worker signed up for a local 10K. She talked about the race with Luisa and something in her started to percolate. Finally giving into curiosity she checked out the website for the run and saw they also had a 5k option. She might not be ready to jump right back into a full 6.2 miles of running but she knew she could do 3.1. So she signed up. If there is ever a gateway drug to running more, it is running a race on the day when others are running further. Before Luisa knew it, she caught the bug again.

Two years later she had completed a half marathon and was running regularly. When her husband was deployed to Iraq, Luisa turned again to running to find solace. She had since moved to Oregon and spent her time running in the dry dusty hills of the Eastern part of the state. For those who don't know the vast wonderfulness of Oregon and think it is all green and rainy, the mountains and foothills of the art of the state, which borders Idaho and Nevada, would come as quite a shock. Luisa decided to step up the normal training and sign up for the Newport Marathon nestled right on the pacific coast of Oregon.

Because of her schedule, being a mom with a husband far away and no one else around to help take care of her children, her entire marathon training regimen came on the revolving belt of a treadmill. If that alone does now show you the intestinal fortitude of a woman hell-bent on making something happen, I do not know what will. Luisa wanted to make this first marathon special. She wanted it to be the culmination of not only this training but of all her training. She wanted it to reflect her decision to recruit the recruiter, of taking on boot camp and of learning how to love something she hated. Of course, the marathon rarely cares what we want it to be. It gives us what it feels like on that day and Luisa was unpleased with her finish time. Running no further than 10 miles on the treadmill didn't exactly help her cause but one must do what they can with what they have.

Nevertheless, it remains her favorite marathon. Struggling through this race, suffering and persevering, Luisa felt it was a mirrored reflection of what she had been through recently. With her husband thousands of miles away in hostile territory Luisa was raising her child on her own. But after five hours and forty-five minutes on the Oregon Coast, she knew no matter how tough life got, or how many times she had to get herself off the floor after feeling as if she could not make it through another day, the finish line was attainable.

Luisa still lives in Eastern Oregon with her two daughters (ten and almost two) and her husband, who still serves in the Armed Forces (US Army). Her running course consists of mountains, rivers, and plenty of farm animals. She has gone back to school and obtained a Master's in School

Psychology. With that in her pocket, she is taking time to raise her toddler the best she can. But her eyes are on the Marines again. This time, however, it is not any recruiters but rather the finish line at the Marine Corps Memorial at the end of the Maine Corps Marathon.

Running the Marine Corps Marathon will be her way to say "Thank you" to the Corps for introducing her to something for which she is eternally indebted. For Luisa, running is the most democratic thing about a country she now calls home. An act as simple and natural as running is forbidden for women in so many parts of the world. If legal, it is at least frowned upon. When Luisa is struggling to go out on a run, she tried to remember how she is afforded so many rights others can only have in dreams. She is also allowed to dream, herself. One of those dreams is to go home to Nicaragua.

Luisa has never been back to the place of her birth. Her father, with whom she had a rather estranged relationship with, hasn't seen her in thirty years. In spite of this, she longs to bridge the gap. She knows her father has a drinking problem, as do many of those in impoverished countries. Ideally, she hopes to go back to her father, who she hears is still a strong man and very proud of her, and take him for a run. Maybe she can even convince him to sign up for a race. Perhaps she can even get him to stop drinking. Perhaps. That might be wishful thinking. But goals are only grabbed by those who dream. She wonders if she would have even tried to dream back in Nicaragua.

Luisa current dream is to run a half-marathon every month for a year in 2014. While doing so she hopes to continue to better her children's lives. She already knows how lucky her daughters are to have so many readily available opportunities. Chances she herself would have never had back in her native country.

She faced down a Marine recruiter because she was told women weren't good enough. She dreamed she could do so much more. Now, her daughters, on the high desert plains of Eastern Oregon, can dream about whatever they please.

14

Breezy Bochenek

We often use the word bravery incorrectly. When people make decisions where there is no choice, bravery is usually not the way their actions should be categorized. What they chose was more a foregone conclusion than it was a decision. Brianne Bochenek, who likes to go by the nickname "Breezy", showed different, but equally as impressive character traits at an early age. Just nine years old, Breezy was told she had cancer.

The rare bone cancer Breezy had is called Osteosarcoma. An aggressive cancer usually found in young children, it can often be treated without any loss of limb initially. However, complications down the road often end up making the decision for the person with the cancer to eventually have surgery to remove the cancer, possible infection and ultimately an appendage. When Breezy was told these statistics and how amputating her leg where the cancer was located would greatly increase her chances of surviving, she weighed her options carefully. Her family was shaken and debating what the right course of action would be. How can such a young person be forced to make such a difficult and life-altering choice? However, for Breezy it was not a choice at all.

Blessed with the straightforwardness of youth, Breezy saw a problem and a set of circumstances which would be the most likely to solve the problem. Her mother and father worried what the correct choice would be and Breezy eased their minds with her matter-of-fact approach. There was one way in which she had the best chance to get on with her life and that was going to be without one of her legs.

Breezy has a wonderfully supportive family. She also lived a rather great life for the first nine years. Children who grow up in those circumstances are not usually the most adept at handling such life-altering decisions. If anything, Breezy's attitude toward her dilemma showed unparalleled poise and intelligence for a child her age. For her, all along there was no choice. She was not being brave in her mind, but rather rational, intelligent and also logical. She now had a solution to a problem that had bothered her for quite some time.

The pain in her leg started in a soccer tournament in 2011. Playing through the pain is what kids do, seemingly impervious to exhaustion and agony. Children tend to want to blend in, and in team sports, not giving your all can be seen as hurting the team. The team is often comprised of your friends and no one wants to let their friends down. So she kept playing.

After the tournament, the pain increased. They visited some doctors and therapists and the initial thoughts were that Breezy's IT band was stretching unnaturally. A routine

X-ray revealed the problem was not so simple. Breezy had cancer.

As a runner, if the cancer called Osteosarcoma sounds familiar, you might be thinking of the inspirational Canadian Terry Fox. After being diagnosed with the disease, Terry also had his leg amputated. After deciding to, at first, run a marathon as a one-legged man, he then wanted to go even bigger. Way bigger. The Marathon of Hope Terry started was a planned run where he would, with just a friend or two in a van, run the entire way across Canada. About halfway across Canada, Terry's cancer returned. He eventually succumbed to the diseases without completing his journey. His legacy survives in Canada today while charity runs continue to raise millions decades after his passing. Breezy hopes, like Terry, she can inspire others with her own battle and with advances in medicine and treatment, she can do so in person for a long time to come.

Being a role model and someone people of all ages will look to for inspiration appears to be a natural thing for Breezy. Her demeanor is amazingly positive especially given the fact that she is not completely out of the woods yet. Her test results remain negative and the news she has received positive, but she knows she must continue her battle. Yet the ease with which she handles a room belies the naturally shy and reserved nature of this young girl. As she gives lectures and TEDtalks about how her diagnosis has changed her life, you do not see fear or dread. Instead, you see a fighter. You see the spirit of a warrior packed into a tiny little body.

When she learned the cancer was in her leg, Breezy simply said they should cut the portion of the leg off which was bad and get her a robot leg. "I wanted a leg like Will Smith's arm in iRobot." When it became clear it would not just be a small sliver of her leg but rather everything below the knee, the importance of this news was not lost on her. Yet she did not shirk from what she felt was necessary. Start the chemotherapy, lose the bad leg and let's get back to life.

Ironically, being dealt such a potentially lethal blow has not lessened the religious faith for either Breezy or her family. They will not be given more than they can handle and with a tight-knit family and a supportive community, they can handle a great deal. Moreover, Breezy doesn't have to rely just on faith and wishes of a better life. She has found real-life examples of those who had dealt with similar problems and came out the other side.

While preparing for the potential surgery, Breezy happened across the story of Sarah Reinertsen. While Sarah's case was a bone disorder and not the same life-threatening cancer Breezy was facing, the end result was the same. Here was a woman athlete competing at the top of her game with only one leg. Breezy's aunt arranged for a phone call just a few weeks before her surgery from Sarah to Breezy. Then after the surgery, Sarah came out to visit Breezy and lend her own spirit and support in person. For Breezy, this was a major turning point in what she wanted to do with the rest of her life. While Sarah was the first woman with a prosthetic to complete an Ironman triathlon in Kona, "perhaps I will be the youngest," Breezy said.

Breezy's family and friends have been stellar as a foundation for her to rebuild herself both during and after her chemo and surgery. When she started her treatments,

Breezy was quick to lose her hair. A decision was made by ten family members that in solidarity, they would all shave their heads as well. Thirty minutes later, bald domes shined under the lights. The number of follicle-challenged people grew to over thirty as many of Breezy's schoolmates followed suit with the razor.

After the surgery and when she was strong enough post-chemo, Breezy began making a plan to get back into sports. She has always enjoyed being able to run but knew it was going to take some time getting used to her prosthetic leg. Trepidation crept in the most when she remembered she had phys. ed. every day. How would she perform? Would the other students be leery of her leg? Was she going to be an outcast?

Fortunately, the children in her sixth grade class were more curious than anything. They had questions about the surgery, how she was handling day-to-day activities and logistical questions. One girl just stood listening to Breezy talk and then gave her a hug. No words came from her lips. Another classmate who had never interacted with Breezy flat out asked her if they could be friends. The innocence and straightforward nature of children shines through even when adults are worried how they will interact.

The Challenged Athletes Foundation has played a big part in Breezy's life. She feels working with CAF will allow her to keep on a career path down the road as a mentor. Already Breezy has done some mentoring of other children, hoping to help them through their own tough times. Sarah Reinertsen's visits and communication with her meant so much she wanted to give back where and how she could.

Breezy feels she has a long life ahead of her and wishes to bring joy to many others along the way. In the meantime, she also wants to take on her own challenges.

Triathlons are her current passion, even though she still loves running by itself. With three separate triathlons under her belt she is eager to get better. Unlike other athletes, Breezy has to conquer more than must the physical limitations of her sport. She has to do more than work on her endurance, strength and skill. Breezy has to overcome the fact that she is missing a leg.

In spite of this difficulty, roughly a year and a half after her amputation, Breezy found herself at the start of the Wildflower Triathlon. Breezy's father Stan (as well as two other siblings) had already been training for a Half Ironman Triathlon. When Breezy said she wanted to compete in a triathlon as well, it was a no-brainer to bring her into the fold. Never mind the fact that the triathlon she wanted to compete in was just ten days away.

When the Wildflower started, her father simply carried Breezy into the water for the open swim start. The rest was up to her. Following her with a camera attached to his head, Stan documented her entire journey. From putting on her running leg after exiting the water to cycling through the hilly bike course to finishing awash with cheers, Breezy moved forward, even if somewhat awkwardly. For this particular race she had to wear an adult-sized prosthetic leg called a Cheetah, seen on many pro Paralympian's. This springy C-shaped prosthetic may be cutting-edge technology but it does not replace having an actual foot. Moreover, learning how to properly run with it on is something that takes a great deal of time. Breezy was trying to master in in a triathlon after only having it for a week and a half.

But Breezy is fine with this learning curve. Even if she cared how ungainly she looked or how long it would take to get back to the way she was, she knows she is alive. She is running. She continues to move forward each day when so many others do not have that option. Breezy is acutely aware of how lucky she is while at the same time she has a long road ahead. She has seen so many other children her age who have it much worse than she does. She simply hopes that in their toughest time, perhaps they too can find someone who lifts their spirits. If she so happens to be the one who can be a beacon for them in their moment of darkness, then that is just all the better.

15

Camille Herron

The sport of running for virtually 99% of all people who participate in it is simply about pushing their limits and having fun. It is folly to think, however, that having fun is mutually exclusive from running hard. The old perception that you never saw a person smiling while running is an insipid rebuttal to running not being something which can be enjoyable. However, even if one is running hard and having fun, rarely will they have to worry about winning a race. Furthermore, an even smaller subset of the population needs never tor concern itself with winning multiple races and qualifying for the Olympic Trials in the marathon. Camille Herron is in that small subset.

We often hear people say, "Well, I just like to have fun" when they discuss their running. This is almost always done with a dismissive wave of the hand to explain why they do not run a certain speed. It removes the need to be competitive or compensates for what they perceive to be a slower than acceptable time for whatever race they were running. This nonchalant attitude also implies that somehow running as fast as you can is neither fun nor enjoyable. Camille Herron has twice made the Olympic Trials as a marathoner, both in 2008 and 2012. Obviously, Camille rarely just shows up to trot a race at a leisurely pace. Yet, few runners have more fun running at any speed than she does.

Herron holds the world record for the fastest marathon run by a woman wearing a superhero costume. Most of the time when people play dress-up for a marathon, their time is thrown out the window. The point is to simply be goofy. Camille ran a 2:48 marathon in a head-to-toe pink Spiderman costume. Her time broke the previous record of a costumed runner (who basically wore regular running apparel with a cape attached to it) by over 20 minutes.

Fast? Check.

Fun? Yep.

Often when runners are having fun in a race, the idea of actually racing is secondary. They are purposefully going much slower than possible. They are stopping to take pictures of a virtually everyone and everything. This irks some and others do not care. The ones who are bothered feel those not racing to their fullest potential are abusing the gift. They feel there is almost an unspoken commitment by runners that they will give everything they have when they toe the line to race.

Camille has shown the two things, running hard and enjoying every minute of it regardless of what clothing you are wearing, can be done simultaneously.

Upon meeting this tall fit blonde, you can immediately tell she is full of energy. She laughs loudly and from the belly button. Her smile is plentiful and she is quite down-to-earth. The genial way in which she handles herself often belies how talented she is and how hard she works to utilize what she has been given. Camille mentions that she understands how being a fast runner is basically a roll of the genetic dice. Furthermore, being able to compete at the highest level can only be done during a small period of time. Knowing how fleeting this set of circumstances is, many find it difficult to simply have fun.

We have come to expect our elite athletes to reflect this stoic nature and often get bothered when they seem to take it too lightly. Usain Bolt celebrating long before he actually finishes a race seems to smack of both showmanship and hubris, like a god unappreciative of his gifts. We, as mortals, do not like to see some people doing what others could never do with such ease. Their semi lackadaisical attitude reminds us how earthbound we are. But being aware of the sacrifices a runner must make to toe the line and all the pain and suffering one must get through to get to the finish doesn't mean a person can't have fun as well. Camille shows you can do both. Few out there bridge that gap between those who run to represent their country and the rest of us simply hoping to get a shiny medal when our hard day's work of running is over.

Her memories of being fast go back a long way. She recalls training for the Presidential Physical Fitness Test in elementary school and being faster than all the others. When she moved onto track in 7th grade she found her stamina increased the longer she ran. She lobbied to be a long distance runner as sprinting simply wasn't her bag. Being so aware of her body, when it is good and when it is ailing, has served her greatly since then.

The distances got longer, the times got faster and eventually Camille found herself qualified for the U.S. Olympic Trials in 2008. However, a stress fracture in her fibula laid-low any plans for her to run to her fullest potential there. Undeterred, Camille treated her first Olympic Trials a spectator of sorts. She still ran in the race but it was more about experiencing the thrill of the electric environment. She knew getting to this race was a huge achievement but finishing it without further injury was the biggest reward. Then she took off time to train and heal, hoping for another chance to prove what she had inside of her.

Fortunately, Camille had the talent and luck to once again qualify for the trials in 2012. This time she returned fit, healthy, and ready to roll. When the day was over, she scorched her previous personal best and ran a time of 2:37:14. She still allowed herself to experience the electric environment, but this time her fitness and health were completely in sync. Anyone lucky enough to have that rare day where everything clicks knows exactly what Camille was feeling when she was able to get in the zone and push the pace as hard as possible. The runners around her moved in time and she used their energy to go as fast as she ever had. Her competitors lifted her, just as they do runners in the middle or back of the back. She was having a blast.

With Camille's knowledge of her ability to run faster the further she goes, it was never a question of if she would run an ultramarathon but when. This is how she found herself in South Africa at the start of the famed Comrades Marathon.

Comrades is actually a misnamed race, at least as far as we know what a marathon is these days. The race dates back to 1921 when any race of a long distance was called a marathon. Closer to 56 miles overall, the race is run in one direction one year and then the opposite the next year. Called the "up" and the "down", both are punishing courses regardless of the distance due to the elevation change throughout. As you can assume, many things can happen over that distance even for the naturally gifted and well trained.

Most ultramarathons, even in this day and age where the numbers are growing exponentially, are small affairs with a few hundred runners at most taking part. But Comrades Marathon is bursting at the seams with nearly 18,000 runners every year. Through a rustic environment from Pietermaritzburg to Durban where the race finally leaves the countryside and villages, the mettle of a runner is tested over hill and dale. Yet, even though she had been in the upper echelon of women runners for most of the race, Camille ultimately suffered what all us mortal runners deal with all the time – a bad day.

Dealing with a stomach virus that she may have shared with her husband (or actually got from him in the first place) Camille became beset with diarrhea. The resulting exertion in the race coupled with dehydration had her collapse with just over 3.5 miles to go. The next thing she knew she was in the emergency room with a fever and potassium/hydration depletion. There are few things scarier than being in the ER in a different country. Camille, however, chalked it up to just one of her many life experiences. She never questioned her training or her methods and just chalked up the bug to the same thing we all chalk up our maladies: bad luck. You realize how fleeting success is and then you move on. Take time to re-assess, make changes as necessary and return to normal life.

Real life for Camille is almost the exact same real life as it is for the rest of us. She is not living what many would think to be the dream of sleeping, eating and running. The plain and simple truth is that even with what she has accomplished her speed is not so great to afford her the opportunity to be one of those select few who can make a living on running. There are few who can do so and even those lucky ones survive on threadbare existence most of the time, which is what makes Camille's efforts all that more impressive.

You see she continues to work full-time as a Research Assistant at the University of Oklahoma Health Sciences Center. She realizes the need to strike a balance with everything she does. There was a brief time when she wasn't working full time. During that period she would normally run between 120-140 miles per week. Today, working full-time she still averages right around 100 miles per week. All told, she devotes 65-70 hours per week to her job and running.

The small sponsors she has mostly cover product and gear. Sometimes she is fortunate enough to win a small purse for a victory here and there. However, the amount of money won pales in comparison to time she puts into her races. But money is not the deciding factor. She simply likes to run. She still has to make sure she is fueling and hydrating adequately at work. At night if she wants to have a good day at work and on her run, she has to get enough sleep. In other words, she is more or less just a faster version of most of us.

She started a blog but wondered if anyone was even reading her stories about overcoming injuries and what she ate. However, as the running community is unlike virtually any other athletic community out there, where we get to hobnob with all but the most reclusive of the elites and sub-elites, Camille soon found she had quite a following.

Messages poured in that brought the entire range of emotions. She realized she could use her ability as a platform for greater good, beyond pursuing personal goals. Becoming more involved with the local running community in Oklahoma City was something she felt was a no-brainer. On a grander scale than just Oklahoma she is doing what she can to affect change in the sport itself. As the Secretary for the Women's Long Distance Running Executive Committee for the USATF, Camille is trying to take on the sport from all fronts.

Too often we assume we know other's thought processes or their motivation. We can see someone who has talent and don't see the hard work or sacrifice that comes with it. What makes Camille special is not just her athletic gifts, but what she is doing to give back to the sport which has given her so much.

That is the essence of being a true elite.

16

Sophia Shi

If you have moved to a country in which you don't speak the language and decided to take on a new course of study in microbiology as an adult student, chances are the idea of running 200 miles straight doesn't seem that imposing. Actually, no that's ridiculous. Running 200 miles is imposing no matter who you are or what you have done. But Sophia Shi seems as likely as anyone to take it all in stride.

As one of nine children growing up in Vietnam, life was far from easy for Sophia. Her father's occupation was tied mostly to the American presence there during the conflict in the 1960s and 1970s. When the last Americans left, so did all the work he had been putting in for many years. He lost his job and because of the specificity of what he had done, lost all the experience that came with it. They struggled to make ends meet with so many mouths to feed.

Her father took odd jobs here and there, including some that were far from safe. While they could not prove it, when her father's health started to fail, they were pretty certain his work in some unclean places had probably contributed if not caused the decline. In order to try and get a better life for themselves, some of Sophia's brothers escaped Vietnam and stole away to America in 1978. Even though she was the second youngest, many duties of being a woman of the house fell upon Sophia. But she always had high hopes for where she could eventually go.

Sophia was an avid reader and devoured anything she could get her hands on. She saw National Geographic magazine articles about Yellowstone National Park. Her eyes would get wide at the thought of seeing such an enormous portion of land where she could freely roam. She dreamed of wandering over the countryside, without fear of being told where she could stay or sleep. No armed men patrolling the streets. No borders to cross. Just mountains and streams and fields.

Unfortunately, while she was still growing up, Sophia's father finally succumbed to his illness. This left the remaining members of her family with a very tough decision. Should they continue to try and squeeze out a living in Vietnam, which seemed rather unlikely, or should they take their chances in America? This was also rather daunting. Seeing little they could do in their own country to make a living, her remaining family members followed her brothers to San Francisco.

Sophia arrived in the city by the bay not even knowing how to say "Hello" in English. But the glittering buildings, soaring nearby mountains, fog and water of the bay area was a dream for her. She might not be able to express it in words just yet, but her eyes spoke volumes.

She soon learned that her degree in economics from her college in Vietnam was worth about as much as the paper it was printed on. Sophia realized if she was going to make it in American she was going to have to start from scratch. Having always been a fan of numbers, she mulled over her options. She thought perhaps molecular biology would be the way to make a living. You know, the easy route.

Learning English was paramount to her survival in this new land but in Sophia's mind, science was an international language. If she had any chance to move ahead in America, it would be through this route. But she couldn't do it without at least learning some English. So at 24 years of age, she started taking classes at a community college. At the same time while she was taking classes, she couldn't neglect the necessities of life such as eating and sleeping. So she began working full-time as well and started to put the pieces together to begin a new life.

Time passed and for a while, things were fairly amazing for Sophia. After putting herself through college, finding a husband and starting a family, Sophia felt like she had it all. She got hired at a Biotech company in California and had her first child. In every way her story could be marked as one of success, except for one: her health.

Soon after her son passed his first birthday, she found herself becoming very sick. She was fatigued constantly and had a complete lack of energy. Her entire body was aching and she felt dizzy all the time. When she finally passed out and was found on the floor one day, she went to the doctor. Here they found Sophia was diabetic. In the time she had been in America, she had put so much effort into learning the language, settling down and doing things right for her family, she forgot to take care of herself. Her lithe figure, sporting roughly 100 pounds, had nearly doubled to 190 pounds. She looked at her son and knew she had to do something to be healthy and be around for him for the long haul.

Looking at herself in the mirror she wanted to cry. She hadn't really thought about what she was doing to her health until she had to poke her finger ten times a day to take blood tests. Sophia wasn't sure how she was going to make a change but she knew she was going to find out how. Internet searches allowed her to find story after story of people who lost hundreds of pounds training for marathons. She figured this would be her path to recovery.

For two months she did little more than walk. This progressed to jogging at a very slow pace for a few miles. She felt like every step had to be a step closer to a better healthier life even though she felt as if she would collapse. Sophia had never so much as done a pushup in her life, let alone go for a three mile run. She wanted to quit every day but still put on her shoes and went out the door. This was about more than just her. This was about her family.

By bettering her diet, running four miles in the morning before work and four miles in the evening after work, she dropped thirty pounds in six months. She also joined a gym and put in time working on strength training as well. It took her five long years but with her hard work she lost nearly seventy-five pounds. She was a completely different person.

What is remarkable about Sophia's road to fitness is she seemed to do everything in moderation. She knew it took years for her to get out of shape and it would therefore probably take years to get back into shape. Too often people want quick fixes and instead of working off the pounds simply go to a plastic surgeon. So this everything in moderation attitude really is a stark contrast to what Sophia decided to do next. Having never run more than ten miles, she wanted to take on the marathon.

In December 2008 she took off from the start of her first marathon, and as you can imagine, fell upon some hard times in the latter miles. She did pull herself together to sneak in under five hours but said she would never do it again. With clarity bestowed upon her after realizing a marathon wouldn't be so bad if she actually did proper training, she found herself half a year later knocking over half an hour off her time. The finishing time was still not what she knew she was capable of doing. Yet at the finish she knew that running would be a part of her life from here on out.

It only took her six more months, and a smattering of marathon races, to finally realize a dream: qualifying for the Boston Marathon. When she hit the 25th mile, she knew she was going to get the time she needed. For over a mile tears welled up in her eyes. Her running career had started at the age of 34 and now she was going to run in the Holy Land of running. Of course, as things tend to go like this, her first Boston Marathon was a tough experience. With a calf injury just two weeks prior to race day, she was hobbled quite a bit. On the day when everyone seemed to have their best Boston Marathon time ever, Sophia had a less than stellar time.

But she bounced back. She had been down the tough road before and would not let a bad marathon time get under her skin. In fact, she wanted to continue to push her boundaries. She wanted to take on distances even longer than the marathon. She knew doing so would take an even tighter focus not just on running but on balancing her entire life. Not only would she have to find the time to get in these workouts, she would have to balance it with her life as a mother, wife and scientists. Sophia wanted to show her friends it could all be done.

She knows it is hard to do all of this and easy for people who do not want to run to make excuses why they cannot. Having a husband who supports her racing schedule is something she does not take for granted. Balancing her duties as a family member and her wants to travel and run can sometimes cause friction. Sophia balances this by continuing to be well organized and efficient person by nature. She keeps her kids on a schedule and she sticks to it as well. With her, less time to be idle means more time to be pursuing all of your dreams. She has down time with her kids and family, going on hikes or watching television but she wants to show them that the way to get something in life is by seizing the reins. If you want something bad enough you will realize the only way it will come to you is if you chase after it.

In that vein, Sophia has chased down eight separate 100-mile finishes in her pursuit of happiness and bliss. Running has been the best therapy for her, giving her a sense of purpose. It has been both a mental and physical challenge, something which helps her in everyday life. She sees the sport as somewhat magical, making her feel better than any drug or fatty food ever could. It challenges her but reminds her if she can take on these long distances and still do so with a smile, there is virtually nothing else she cannot do. This, of course, leads us to the 200-mile run mentioned above.

The fall in the Lake Tahoe region is absolutely stunning. Who are we kidding? It is always stunning in Tahoe. But no vista, regardless of how stunning, can prepare you for running 200 miles. Entering into this race, Sophia had no designs on winning. She simply hoped to finish under the 100-hour cutoff. Following a course which circumnavigated Lake Tahoe high in the Sierra Nevada Mountains, the race would be a true test of everything she had put herself through. Her difficult life in Vietnam. Taking on a new country and a new language. Dropping unhealthy weight so she could actually be around for her children's future. Tackling the marathon distance and beyond. All of that was leading to this moment.

When she crossed the finish line with just 101 minutes to spare, she felt both destroyed and invincible. She found it hard to put into words how she could be so absolutely bereft of energy yet feel like there was nothing she could not do, all at the same time. Only 60 people finished the course in the provided time and she was not the last one (Koichi Takeishi, a 51 year old man from Japan made the cutoff by *four seconds*.) Even if she had been last, the feat itself was amazing. Sophia has shown how barriers can be simply the stepping stones we use to get to bigger and better things. We can see the hurdles in front of us as those that will stop us, or those that propel us forward.

Sophia prefers to propel. In fact, just four days after she finished the Tahoe 200, Sophia once again qualified for the Boston Marathon at a high altitude race in Utah.

She still gets tears in her eyes.

17

Monika Allen

Often those who get the spotlight thrust upon them do not get to choose the when or why. They are not looking for attention and when they do get it, it is rarely for what they would like. Taking that rare moment of fame or attention and turning it for good if what makes the few fortunate enough to do so stand out amongst their peers. Monika Allen did just that sort of turning.

Many of those who know Monika Allen might not even know her name. But they assuredly know her as the person SELF Magazine decided had an outfit on they didn't like. Unfortunately for SELF, the outfit was being worn to bring awareness to her battle with brain cancer. *Cue the Price is Right loser horn.*

This entire fiasco started when Monika excitedly received an email from SELF magazine asking for permission to use a photo that showed her running the LA marathon dressed as Wonder Woman. In addition to her superhero outfit she happened to also be donning a tutu. This particular marathon was right in the middle of Monika's chemotherapy and was a celebration of her spirit and tenacity. The tutu?

Well, she made the tutu herself. Her company Glam Runners makes them and donates the money to Girls on the Run (GOTR), a charity that sponsors exercise and confidence-building programs for young girls. Monika says she's raised about $5,600 for the nonprofit by making about 2,000 tutus over the past three years. Not exactly world-changing but without a doubt a wonderful gesture, on Monika's part. However, when the picture appeared in SELF, it had the following caption.

"A racing tutu epidemic has struck NYC's Central Park, and it's all because people think these froufrou skirts make you run faster. Now, if you told us they made people run from you faster, maybe we would believe it."

The slight irony of this statement is a few years ago, if it was said casually by someone not putting it into print, Monika might have laughed at it. As a gymnast and cheerleader growing up, Monika didn't have much time or desire to be a runner. Seeing someone dressed in silly garb in a race might have been reason enough for her to run away from them. It took a roommate in college dragging her to a 10k for her to even think about running. Wearing a cotton hooded-sweatshirt, carrying a Walkman and running in the pouring rain was Monika's first race experience.

It is a small miracle she even made it to the starting line of this race. A casual smoker who thought she would quit before the race started (she did not), Monika continued to smoke on and off for a few years. Since she wasn't running much and wasn't even doing gymnastics anymore, her need for lung capacity was not that high. She thought there was little wrong with a pack of smokes here and there. Only after taking a job in Phoenix where she began working for an oral cancer screening company, did she finally come to her senses. But not right away. Cancer is for other people.

It took some time after her move and her new job for her to realize where she was putting herself. She began to have asthma attacks on a more frequent basis. In hindsight, Monika likens these more to an allergic reaction to her cat than anything to do with smoking. But the shortage of breath and the feeling as if someone was sitting on her chest drove the point home. Running in a 5k, which benefitted cancer research, was the ah-ha moment she needed. Smoking was killing her. She promptly stopped and put the disgusting habit behind her in 2004. A few months later she challenged her new clearer lungs with a half marathon in Phoenix. Feeling like a superhero because of her new greater lung capacity, she signed up for even bigger challenges. In June of 2006, she took on the 26.2 miles offered at the San Diego Marathon.

Over the course of the next few years, Monika enjoyed the life of the average runner. Pushing her boundaries and shooting for PRs, she pursued new horizons. She had moved to San Diego, raced on the weekends, explored the roads in her new home and did what she could to stay fit. Yet in spite of her fitness she was experiencing headaches. These were not run of the mill aches and pains. They were blinding headaches where she found herself needing to sit down when they throbbed. When she moved around in any capacity the pain only got worse. She simply figured she was depriving herself of sleep and needed to get more rest. She had never been big on relaxing or taking it easy. Maybe some solid shuteye for a few days would remedy the situation.

However, medicating with some aspirin and rest never did solve the problem. She realized she needed to see a professional. Painkillers were prescribed by a doctor to dull the pain. However, even if the pain was dulled for a bit, Monika knew there was a reason she was brought to her knees by this searing pain in her head. Masking it was not helping her find the root of the problem. Perhaps it was a slipped disk in her back. Maybe it was something else she didn't have the expertise to figure out. When even the prescription painkillers did not ease the pain she knew she had to do more.

She scheduled an appointment with a neurologist. He more or less brushed off her concerns and ignored her description of the pain. He wasn't aware this was a woman who suffered through the pain of 26.2 miles at a time. She was not one who easily complained of pain. If only to possibly placate her, the doctor begrudgingly ordered some tests be done for Monika.

A few days after her tests she received a call from the doctor's office. No one seemed to be too anxious to speak to her but said she would need to come speak to her physician about the results. As such she wasn't all too worried. Upon meeting the doctor he displayed the same horrible bedside manner he had when he dismissed her initial pain.

"It's not good."

Monika was told she had a brain tumor. The blasé nature with which her physician gave her the news made her think it was a practical joke at first. Soon it dawned on her that he was not joking. She understood the need to be told this news in a straightforward manner but the news she had something growing inside her head simply floored her.

At first she did not know what to do. How does someone react to such news? Soon, however, she knew what she had to do. She scheduled surgery to get what needed to be done as soon as possible. Before long she had a shunt placed in her head to release the fluid from around her brain. Without this device the pressure would have increased and crushed her brain.

While doing this procedure and getting ready for what was to follow, Monika prepared herself the best way she knew how: by reading. Looking back she realized what she was doing with regards to preparation is what runners do when they are getting ready for a marathon. They make a plan, check the elevation, find out where the aid stations are and then finally they run. However, this time, instead of trying to set a new personal best, she was planning for her life.

In her preparation, she happened across a blog about fertility preservation. Given the chemotherapy she was about to go through, she realized she might need to look into having her eggs harvested and frozen. Then it hit her that no one had mentioned this to her at her doctor's office. Why hadn't they informed her, a youngish female who was healthy otherwise and married with no children that she might wish to think about the future? This was when her doctor, once again without much couth, told her that her brain tumor is inoperable. Technically, this means she is, in her own words, doomed.

Undeterred, Monika figured she would do what she had to do to make this tumor take her down swinging. For a year she underwent chemo. In addition, she decided to undertake the supreme challenge of training for and running a marathon while she simultaneously poisoned herself from the inside out. Then she thought she might as well do two separate marathons. This brings us back to the SELF Magazine article.

Monika first learned about the picture when her husband saw the article on his iPad. At first they were happy to see her in a magazine, as would anyone. Then her husband looked closer. "Honey, you might want to check out the caption." Monika checked out the magazine and was completely stunned. She posted the picture and caption on her own website. She wasn't necessarily trying to attack SELF but rather show that sometimes being asked to appear in a magazine might not be all that it is cracked up to be. But her post went viral.

For Monika, this snafu by SELF, while not so great at first has led to many unexpected outcomes. First and foremost, her support for GOTR through her tutu making side-business has skyrocketed. Normally, if she really puts her nose to the grindstone, she can make between 10-20 tutus in a week. After her story hit the news she was getting 40 orders an hour. After just a few days she had to take down the order sheet. She simply couldn't hope to keep up with the demand. She loved that so many people wanted to support her but she was not a business set up to handle such a high demand. Instead, she sent people to the GOTR site directly saying, if you want to help, then do so here.

Also, name recognition for GOTR grew because of her involvement with the organization. More and more people were hearing about GOTR for the first time and inquiring how they could either join a chapter in their area or help start a new one. The SELF magazine editor herself not only apologized for the piece but also made a donation to GOTR. In addition she made a separate donation to research labs dealing with the type of brain cancer that Monika has. In the end, the slight embarrassment has led to some wonderful things in the areas Monika holds most dear. However, this entire string of events makes Monika ponder sometimes.

She is happy her condition brought light to both the battle she is fighting and the causes she runs for but what if she did not have a brain tumor? What if the post had not gone viral? Would SELF Magazine still have apologized? Why did it take someone on the extreme end of the spectrum to make the magazine think twice about taking pot shots at runners? (SELF Magazine has since taken the offending section out of their magazine.) Shouldn't it be a good business model to simply make fun of no one out there struggling to better themselves? Has our culture gotten so crass, so starved for stories in the 24/7 news cycle that anything that gets clicks on a website is worth publishing, regardless of who it may harm? It is wonderful SELF apologized for positing the picture and caption but the fact remains if they had any business acumen at all, they had to. There was no choice here.

Undoubtedly others have probably written into the magazine about similar complaints. SELF claims to hold itself above the cattiness of other similar magazines. This time, however, the magazine mocked a woman running in apparel made specifically to benefit an organization that is meant to empower and lift up young females. Almost accidentally it brought to light how women struggle with issues regarding what they wear and how they look. While men often bear the brunt for placing unrealistic standards of women, it only takes a second to see that this sort of shaming so to speak is intra-gender. Women can be their genders' own worst enemy in the fight for acceptance of their own bodies. Monika is hoping she can help out an end to in fighting.

She knows her days left on this planet are short in number. Monika is basically hoping she has come around right when medicine and science are coming together to fix her problem. She is praying she will be in that group of people who were the first to know that brain cancer is not immediately fatal. In her best estimate she feels she has about ten years to fight this tumor before she will finally succumb to it. Presently it has been about eight months since her last round of chemo. The tumor in her head is stable. She gets an MRI very two months just to see how everything is going. She feels fit and healthy. Her running has not suffered much and her headaches have all but disappeared. For Monika it is just extremely eerie to feel just fine but know she has a time bomb ticking. But if anything, this dilemma has given her a new perspective.

She hopes to use her time left to make changes that need to be made. She wants to do what she can to lift up women, give them support when they need it most, and stop the useless squabbles. Before she became a headline, Monika was already fighting in her own small way. Now, because of a nasty caption, she has a larger platform. She promises not to waste this opportunity.

Her actions are reflections of her knowledge that tomorrow may easily be her last day. She must do everything she can to immediately affect change lest she never has a chance to see it take form. Monika knows it took something horrible in her life for her to really seize this opportunity but she does not shirk from the chance to do more. Hopefully, while she fights, the rest of us can see the same thing and not wait until it is too late.

18

Where can we go from here?

What can we expect from women runners in the future? Your guess is as good as anyone else's. Thirty years ago, no one could have seen that women would be the dominant participants in races in the United States, comprising over half of all finishers. Women drive the economics of the sport from participation to apparel to fund-raising. Every aspect of the sport is intimately woven into the fabric of the runners who not too long ago weren't even allowed to participate.

Predictions are often a fool's game. One only need look at the Deccan Records representative who rejected the Beatles over Brian Pole and the Tremeloes under the assumption that "guitar groups are on the way out." Yet it does not take a crystal ball to see that running canno function without women being part of it.

There are ideas and some science in which seems posit that women might be better suited for the ultra-lo distances of running. The composition of their bodies and way they handle pain and endurance might be able to w down the naturally stronger male body. The gap is ind closing between the two genders in that part of the sport, even if it hasn't come to fruition yet. But the idea is there.

Women already head some of the biggest positions in the sport with the likes of Mary Wittenberg being the President and CEO of the New York Road Runners in which helms the New York City Marathon. Female-specific running stores, magazines and clothing lines are constantly popping up to fill the needs and wants of women runners.

With so much untapped potential and innovation to come from a gender which had so little input for so long, making an accurate guess on where women in the sport of running will be in the future is difficult. But it will no doubt be fantastic.

to
ng
he
ear
eed